The following chapters were adapted from and reprinted by permission of *Medical Self-Care* magazine, P.O. Box 1000, Pt. Reyes, CA 94956; "Red Pepper, the Hot Healer" ("Red Pepper Is Hot," September/October 1989); "Echinacea: A Flower with Power" (Echinacea: Wonder Herb," November/December 1989); "The Right Way to Get Your 'A' " ("Vitamin A: Bugs Bunny Was Right," September/October 1989). "The Mood/Music Connection" and "Can We Talk?" were adapted from *Healthy Pleasures*, by Robert Ornstein and David Sobel. Copyright © 1989 by Robert Ornstein and David Sobel. Reprinted by permission of Addison-Wesley Publishing Co.

Prevention magazine is a registered trademark of Rodale Press, Inc.

Printed in the United States of America on acid-free paper ∞

If you have any questions or comments concerning this book, please write:
Rodale Press
Book Reader Service
33 East Minor Street
Emmaus, PA 18098

ISBN 0–87857–913–3 hardcover

Distributed in the book trade by St. Martin's Press

2 4 6 8 10 9 7 5 3 1 hardcover

Contributors to
The *Natural Healing and Nutrition Annual 1991*

Writers: *Kim Anderson, Pamela Boyer, Jan Bresnick, Jan Eickmeier, Sharon Ferguson, Sid Kirchheimer, Steven Lally, Cemela London, Michael McGrath, Gloria McVeigh, Gale Malesky, Joe Mullich, Cathy Perlmutter, Violette Phillips, Andrew Roblin, Jean Rogers, Porter Shimer, Maggie Spilner, Susan Zarrow*
Production Editor: *Jane Sherman*
Book Design: *Peter A. Chiarelli*
Cover Design: *Darlene Schneck*
Copy Editor: *Candace Levy*
Associate Research Chief, *Prevention* magazine: *Pam Boyer*
Office Manager: *Roberta Mulliner*
Office Personnel: *Barbara Bach, Karen Earl-Braymer*

Contents

Newsfront

Nutritional Healing Strategies

Your Healthy Heart

Super-Nutrient News

Eat Right for Life

Natural Tranquilizers

Maximum Immunity

Shape Up for Health

Mind/Body Healing Strategies

Be Your Personal Best

Body-Care Updates

Special Supplement

SUPPLEMENTS AND COMMON SENSE

Some of the reports in this book give accounts of the professional use of nutritional supplements. While food supplements are in general quite safe, some can be harmful if taken in very large amounts. Be especially careful not to take more than these commonsense limits:

Vitamin A	2,000 I.U.
Vitamin B_6	50 mg
Vitamin D	400 I.U.
Selenium	100 mcg

NOTICE

The information and ideas in this book are meant to supplement the care and guidance of your physician, not to replace it. The editor cautions you not to attempt diagnosis or embark upon self-treatment of serious illness without competent professional assistance. An increasing number of physicians are ready to cooperate with clients who want to improve their diet and lifestyle; if you are under professional care or taking medication, we suggest discussing this possibility with your doctor.

Introduction:
Spin the Wheel of Health

What do you think this still-new decade will bring? Health fads have come and gone, yet most people have successfully made some important lifestyle changes—whether it's buckling up, trimming down, eating more vegetables, or cutting cholesterol. (Will anyone be smoking by 2000?) Only one thing is certain. Some health facts will still be standing and others will be turned on their heads.

Even in this age of uncertainty, I have come to know several things: I feel better when I eat light, simple meals and exercise regularly. Nature has a bounty of secret weapons to deter illness. And the more I know about them and new health discoveries, the better health decisions I can make.

And the more information *you* have, the better off you will be when you want to outpace illness or stay vital. That's why we've packed this annual with clear, fascinating, easy-to-use, and up-to-date information. We've scoured thousands of current scientific journals, interviewed hundreds of physicians to get the inside story on major breakthroughs and new discoveries, and taken the time to double-check every fact. We'll tell you about the newest, smartest—and safest—nutrition advice and natural techniques to heal your body and mind. Along with you and your physician, we can form a strong circle of health that will help you improve your chances of health success.

I hope you enjoy it. I think you'll find the wheel of health will spin a lot smoother the more you know about and use nature's secret health weapons.

Here's to your health and happiness!

Heidi Rodale

Newsfront

KICK BACK AND KNOCK OUT INFECTIONS

Taking some time to mellow out is a good prescription for stress-related health problems. Now research hints that there may be an unexpected bonus: Regular relaxation may help you avoid infections.

Doctors at the University of Pittsburgh School of Medicine measured the activity of natural killer (NK) cells, immune cells that fight infection and malignancy, in 106 healthy people. NK cell activity is a measure of the ability of NK cells to destroy target cells in a laboratory test.

About one-third of the people studied had NK activity that was below average (but still in the normal range). These people reported significantly more colds, flu, and other infectious illnesses over the six months of the study.

The most illnesses occurred in people with low NK cell activity who were younger than 30 and reported a more intense and disruptive level of stress.

This research builds on previous findings, suggesting that relaxation therapy can boost NK cell activity, says Sandra M. Levy, Ph.D., associate professor of psychiatry and medicine at the University of Pittsburgh. It holds particular promise for certain groups of young people who are notorious for developing infections: military recruits and medical students and interns, for example. It's possible, she says, that if they use relaxation therapy, they can raise their NK cell activity and thereby reduce their risk of developing infections. Proof positive, however, is still a long way off.

If you're interested in giving it a try, there is a wide variety of effective relaxation techniques, she says, such as systematic relaxation and self-hypnosis.

1

WALKERS TAKE AN ACTIVE STEP AGAINST CANCER

If you walk for exercise, you may be getting more than you bargained for. Sure, plenty of walking exercise can lower blood pressure, reduce your risk of heart disease, keep bones and muscles strong, and help raise your spirits. But you may also be getting an extra benefit from walking: protection against cancer.

Several studies can now be added to the stack of evidence that points to a link between exercise and reduced cancer risk, though a cause-and-effect relationship hasn't yet been proved.

In one study, researchers examined and interviewed over 8,000 Japanese men living in Hawaii. Those who were moderately or highly active had only half to three-quarters the colon cancer risk of those who were sedentary. The relative risk of colon cancer also decreased as resting heart rate decreased. Lower resting heart rate is one result of regular aerobic exercise, such as brisk walking (*American Journal of Epidemiology*).

Several years ago, a study at Harvard found a lower risk of breast cancer (and other reproductive cancers) in 5,000 women who were athletes during their college years. In a follow-up study of the women, researchers found the prevalence of other cancers was lower as well. Cancers of the digestive system (including the colon), thyroid, bladder, lungs, and blood system were all less common in former athletes (*Medicine and Science in Sports and Exercise*).

One theory: According to Rose Frisch, Ph.D., associate professor of population sciences at the Harvard Center for Population Studies, athletes may have better "immune surveillance." That is, their immune system may be more active against cancer.

This is supported by laboratory research. Physical activity has been linked with increased activity of natural killer (NK) cells, immune components that can destroy tumor cells. One study from Denmark found significantly higher NK cell activity in bicycle racers compared to untrained men who did not paricipate in sports regularly (*International Journal of Sports Medicine*).

MICROWAVE POPCORN: WATCH THE CALORIES

You may have heard popcorn makes a good, low-fat snack. Prepared in an air popper, 1 cup contains only 27 calories, a trace of fat, and almost no sodium. Popping in vegetable oil and adding salt ups the ante to 41 calories, 1.4 grams of fat, and 175 milligrams of sodium.

Microwave popcorn is another story. It's often processed with fats, oils, and salt. Most brands checked in a survey by *Prevention* have three times the fat of plain or oil-popped popcorn. One cup can pack up to 60 calories and 63 milligrams of sodium, even before you salt it.

Not all microwave popcorn brands sport these unflattering figures, though. Orville Redenbacher's, for example, is comparable to air-popped popcorn in calories. (And microwave popcorn generally has fewer calories, less fat, and less sodium than potato chips.)

The bottom line: As with other products, read microwave popcorn labels before you buy.

MIGRAINES YIELD TO COLD PRESSURE

The pain of migraine headaches may be caused in part by an increase in blood flow to the scalp and brain. So for years migraine sufferers have applied cold, damp washcloths to their head. Cold decreases blood flow and may help reduce migraine pain.

That's part of the theory behind the Champ Coldwrap, a cold pack in an elastic bandage with a Velcro closure. It's also thought that the compression provided by the elastic and Velcro may reduce blood flow and relieve migraines.

In one study, when used at the start of a migraine, or when headaches were of dull intensity, the Coldwrap applied for 30 minutes relieved pain somewhat in 29 of 45 migraineurs. Although the study is unpublished and inconclusive (it didn't determine whether a cold washcloth would have had the same effect or whether subjects' expectations of pain relief may have done the trick), previous studies support the idea that cold and pressure may help alleviate migraines.

Coldwrap sells in drugstores and supermarkets for about $7.

FISH OIL MAY REEL IN HYPERTENSION

For years, studies have suggested a link between fish oil and lowered blood pressure. Now scientists at Vanderbilt University offer the first solid evidence that one may indeed exist.

For four weeks, they studied 32 mildly hypertensive men. Eight of the men took 50 milliliters of fish oil per day (equivalent to 2 pounds of mackerel), 8 took 10 milliliters of fish oil, 8 took 50 milliliters of safflower oil (less than $3\frac{1}{2}$ tablespoons), and another 8 took 50 milliliters of a mix of oils approximating those in our diet. To account for any non-fish-oil changes in blood pressure, scientists measured pressure for four weeks before and after the oil regimens.

As usual in such studies, almost everybody's blood pressure fell at first. Once they started the oil regimens, though, only men taking the 50 milliliters of fish oil recorded a significant drop.

After the oil regimen ended, pressure in the group taking the high dose returned to prestudy levels, exactly as it should if fish oil were really responsible for the drop in blood pressure (*New England Journal of Medicine*).

Researchers also noticed that after fish-oil intake, there was a transitory increase in prostacyclins, substances that may indirectly or directly lower blood pressure, says Howard R. Knapp, M.D., Ph.D., the study's head researcher.

Although this research is promising, further study is necessary to confirm the results and to determine fish oil's safety and usefulness. High doses of fish oil can have significant side effects such as prolonged bleeding time. Stay tuned.

LOW POTASSIUM LINKED TO HIGH BLOOD PRESSURE

Over the years, population studies have linked the prevalence of high blood pressure with dietary intake of potassium: the more potassium, the less hypertension. Now an experiment at Temple University School of Medicine in Philadelphia suggests potassium depletion may actually cause high blood pressure, something population studies could not establish.

Researchers fed ten men with normal blood pressure two diets that were identical except for one thing: One provided normal amounts of potassium, while the other was low in the mineral. Sodium intake was kept at the men's usual levels. The men spent nine days on each diet.

The average arterial pressure, a measurement that takes into account both systolic and diastolic pressure, did not change during normal potassium intake. But it increased from an average of 90.9 to 95 while the men ate a low-potassium diet. Sodium and fluid retention also rose (*New England Journal of Medicine*).

G. Gopal Krishna, M.D., the head researcher, speculates that diets insufficient in potassium may cause the body to retain sodium. Over time, this continuous high sodium level may induce hypertension, he says. (Sodium has been implicated in hypertension.)

These findings need to be confirmed. But for now, the Committee on Dietary Allowances' estimated safe and adequate intake (1,875 to 5,625 milligrams per day) of potassium is a good guide to follow, says Dr. Krishna. A medium-size banana contains 451 milligrams of potassium and ½ cup of lima beans, 485 milligrams. Other good sources include melon and potatoes.

VEGETABLES: LEAN AND MEAN CANCER FIGHTERS

Meat eaters may seem fierce, but when it comes to fighting off cancer, vegetarians may pack more punch.

Many studies of large populations have suggested that people who eat vegetarian diets have a lower risk of developing cancer. But scientists don't yet know why.

There are three theories: (1) that vegetarian diets contain more anticancer agents, or that meat-containing diets contain more procancer agents, such as saturated fat; (2) that vegetarian fare is lower in calories, which has been associated with reduced cancer risk in some studies; or (3) that vegetarians have a more active immune system. All three may contribute, and a study from researchers in West Germany adds some preliminary evidence for the latter.

They found vegetarians' white blood cells to be twice as deadly to tumor cells as those of meat eaters. That is, the same volume of white blood cells killed twice as many tumor cells. The researchers speculate vegetarians may have more natural killer (NK) cells among their white cells, more ferocious NK cells, or both (*Nutrition and Cancer*).

RELAXATION MAY HELP DIABETES

Diabetes prescription of the future: Relax after every meal. At least, that could conceivably be the case if preliminary evidence holds true.

Researchers at the Duke University Medical Center studied the effects of relaxation in 20 people with Type II (non-insulin-dependent) diabetes. All were given proper diabetes education and medication. But half also received training in the antistress therapy called "progressive muscle relaxation" and were told to practice it twice a day.

Blood tests to assess glucose tolerance (the body's ability to properly metabolize sugar, which is impaired in diabetics), were taken at the beginning and end of the 24-week study. The experimental group was told to practice their relaxation exercise during the final test.

Only the patients who received relaxation training improved glucose tolerance—by an average of 20 percent. Some even improved by 30 percent, the researchers report.

"It may be important for people with Type II diabetes to remain relaxed after meals in order to improve their diabetes control," says Richard S. Surwit, Ph.D., professor of medical psychology and associate professor of medicine at Duke. Dr. Surwit and his colleagues plan a follow-up study to determine if relaxation can affect long-term control in diabetes.

If you have Type II diabetes, you might want to talk to your doctor about using relaxation techniques. "It can't hurt," says Dr. Surwit. "At the very least, it should reduce anxiety, which is a common symptom of the disorder." (Current research indicates that relaxation techniques are not as useful in Type I diabetes.)

BLOCK THE SUN AND VITAMIN D?

Sunscreens block harmful ultraviolet rays. Of course. At the same time, sunscreens may also block what dermatologists say is the only known benefit of sun exposure: our skin's production of vitamin D.

So says a preliminary study (*Archives of Dermatology*). Scientists recruited 20 white people, average age 65, in Springfield, Illinois, and Philadelphia, Pennsylvania. For more than a year, all applied sunscreen with a sun-protection factor (SPF) of 15 to exposed skin before going outside. Scientists also recruited a similar group of 20 people who didn't use sunscreen.

In summer, when synthesis of vitamin D from sunlight should peak in these geographic areas, both groups gave blood samples. Blood from people who didn't use sunscreen had normal vitamin D levels. Sunscreen users didn't do so well. Most were within the normal range but on the low side. Two showed signs of vitamin D deficiency.

Vitamin D deficiency causes one disease with two names. In children, it's called rickets; in adults, osteomalacia. Children's bones don't form properly; adults' soften. Vitamin D deficiency has also been linked to the hip fracture disease, osteoporosis. Low-but-normal vitamin D values may also be cause for concern—particularly in summer, when we should store lots of vitamin D to get us through the dark days of winter.

The sunscreen studied was made with para-aminobenzoic acid (PABA). Sunscreens made with other substances likely have the same effect. They, too, absorb the wavelengths of ultraviolet light we use for vitamin D production.

Lower SPFs probably don't help, either. An SPF as low as 8 completely stops vitamin D production.

This doesn't mean we should stop using sunscreen. First, the benefits of sunscreen in preventing sunburn, skin cancer, and other hazards outweigh the risks of not using it. Second, this study is small and preliminary. It didn't measure actual sun exposure or dietary vitamin D.

Still, it can't hurt most of us who use sunscreen to get the Recommended Dietary Allowance of vitamin D: 200 international units per day. Good sources include vitamin D–fortified milk, mackerel, salmon, and fortified breakfast cereals.

But thin, older white women (most at risk for osteoporosis) who avoid sun exposure or use sunscreens extensively—because of, say, fair or sun-damaged skin or a history of skin cancer—should consult their doctor. For them, increasing their vitamin D intake through vitamin D–rich foods, or in some cases, supplements, may be the simplest preventive step.

THE PROTEIN/BREAST CANCER CONNECTION

You may be aware of the association between a high-fat diet and increased risk of breast cancer. Now findings suggest that a diet high in saturated fat and animal protein may also have a link.

Scientists in Italy interviewed 250 women, almost every breast cancer patient in the province of Vercelli. They also interviewed 499 similar women without breast cancer.

Patients reported higher consumption of whole milk, high-fat cheese, butter, meat, and eggs. In fact, women with the highest intake of saturated fat or animal protein had two to three times the risk of breast cancer as those on low-fat diets (*Journal of the National Cancer Institute*).

Based on these data, the researchers who conducted the study suggest that following current dietary recommendations, which emphasize low-fat dairy products and non-meat sources of protein (such as beans and fish), may help protect against breast cancer. Start by switching to skim milk, limiting high-fat cheese to no more than five slices per week and replacing butter with margarine or olive oil, says study leader Paolo Toniolo, M.D., assistant professor of environmental medicine at New York University Medical Center.

EASY WORKOUTS MAY EASE ARTHRITIS

Many doctors used to tell their patients with arthritis not to exercise. Not anymore. Accumulating research shows that aerobic exercise—the kind that gives the heart a workout—helps people with arthritis.

According to a summary of studies on the subject, aerobic exercise actually reduces joint pain. Other benefits: It increases strength and aerobic capacity (our ability to take in air and circulate blood). And it may improve more subjective concerns, such as mood and social activity (*The Physician and Sportsmedicine*).

If your doctor approves, try walking, dancing, swimming, or if knee disease isn't severe, bicycling. (Stationary bikes are best unless you ride on very flat terrain.)

A good place to start is with the Arthritis Foundation's People with Arthritis Can Exercise (PACE) program. You can get the program's home videotapes, or you can participate in a class taught by trained instructors. Contact your local Arthritis Foundation chapter or write to P.O. Box 19000, Atlanta, GA 30326. Ask for brochure number 9763. You can also request brochure number 9704, which tells how to exercise safely. Both brochures are free.

MIND OVER TOOTHACHE

"When I snap my fingers, your teeth will be totally free of pain." That's the gist of a possible treatment for people with painful tooth-root sensitivity.

These patients feel pain when their teeth are exposed to various stimuli: hot or cold beverages, tooth brushing, or mouthwash, for example. About 5 to 10 percent of the population experience this problem. Often, it causes them to alter their diet.

Dentists in the U.S. Air Force Dental Corps tested the effectiveness of hypnosis in eight patients who had suffered from hypersensitive teeth for an average of $4\frac{1}{2}$ years. The dentists induced hypnosis, then told each patient that he could tolerate or ignore pain on either the right or left side of his mouth. The other side served as the "control" for comparison. The patients were then "awakened." The treatment was repeated one week later, and the patients rated their level of pain daily.

Three weeks after the last treatment, seven of the eight patients rated the treatment side as having a greater decrease in the amount of pain. Pain was eliminated completely in four patients, and all eight improved significantly over the test period.

Four of the patients were unable to confine the effect of hypnotherapy to one side of the mouth. At last check, the good results had lasted six months, according to Clifford B. Starr, D.M.D., one of the researchers.

Hypnosis is not the first choice for therapy, says Robert B. Mayhew, D.M.D., Ph.D., another of the researchers, especially since these results must be considered preliminary until proved in a larger study. But it remains a promising last resort for people who don't find relief with standard treatments: desensitizing toothpaste, fluoride gel applications, and the combined use of fluoride and electric currents.

And because hypnosis can mask pain that may provide a clue toward accurate diagnosis, it's best used when the dentist is totally familiar with a patient's dental history.

For referral to a dentist in your area who practices hypnosis, send a self-addressed stamped envelope to the American Society of Clinical Hypnosis, 2250 E. Devon Ave., Suite 336, Des Plaines, IL 60018.

HIGH-FIBER DIET SHRINKS COLON POLYPS

A fiber of good news in the fight against cancer: Adding wheat bran to the diet may shrink precancerous polyps in the lower intestine, reducing the risk of colon and rectal cancer, a study suggests.

Researchers at the New York Hospital-Cornell Medical Center in New York City studied 58 people with familial polyposis. People with this inherited condition develop polyps in the colon and rectum that often develop into cancer.

The study participants were asked to eat two servings of cereal from unmarked boxes every day for four years. Half were given a cereal high in wheat bran, an insoluble fiber (for a total of 22.5 grams of fiber a day). The other half were given a low-fiber look-alike.

In addition, half the people in the high-fiber group and half of the low-fiber group were given supplements of vitamins C and E. And all the participants' diets were analyzed for fat intake. The patients were examined every three months.

In those people who carefully followed the high-fiber diet, polyps were more likely to shrink in both size and number than to grow. The low-fiber group had no such benefit. While there were hints that vitamins C and E were also beneficial, the results were not statistically significant. A higher fat intake was associated with more polyps, however.

The study doesn't conclusively prove that wheat bran fiber can inhibit cancer in these people. But "substantial evidence strongly suggests that if you can prevent polyps you can ultimately prevent cancer," says Jerome J. De-Cosse, M.D., Ph.D., the study's head researcher.

Doctors don't know exactly how bran works, he says, but it may dilute carcinogens in the bowel, reducing exposure of its inner walls to the damaging substances.

While the study looked only at people with familial polyposis, Dr. DeCosse believes "it is likely that a high-insoluble-fiber, low-fat diet will benefit the general population." Previous studies have suggested that people who eat a high-fiber diet are less likely to develop colorectal cancer.

This is the first study to find that an ordinary food can inhibit a premalignant condition.

BORON AND BRAIN WAVES

A researcher at the Grand Forks Human Nutrition Research Center in North Dakota suggests that boron may have a role in the brain.

Fifteen people over age 45 had earlier participated in a study that showed a possible link between boron and bone health. James G. Penland, Ph.D., studied the same group, who spent 14 days on a diet with adequate boron, 63 days on a low-boron diet, and 49 days back on the boron-replete diet. He found changes in the electrical impulses in their brain that indicate a possible decrease in mental alertness while they were on the low-boron diet. These effects are identical to those he found in a study of laboratory rats.

To a certain extent, those changes happen naturally as people age, says Dr. Penland. "But we saw that same pattern exaggerated when the people were on the low-boron diet. So perhaps, combined with some other stresses on the system, low boron might result in poorer performance of a task."

But the significance of this finding goes beyond boron's possible effect on mental alertness. "This is one of the first pieces of data to show that by altering the amount of boron in your diet, you can have an effect on something functional; in this case, the electrical activity of the brain," says Dr. Penland. "It's too early to know for sure, but it looks as though boron will turn out to be an essential nutrient for humans."

You can easily get all the boron you need by eating a healthful diet containing apples, pears, grapes, nuts, prunes, raisins, dates, tomatoes, and red peppers. That's the best approach, as large doses of the mineral can be toxic.

VITAMIN C KEEPS YOUR LUNGS BREATHING EASY

If you eat plenty of foods rich in vitamin C, you can breathe easier—for two reasons. One, because those foods (fruit, melons, and vegetables) contribute amply to a healthful diet. And two, because vitamin C in the diet has been linked to fewer lung problems.

In a study of over 9,000 people, those whose diet provided 100 milligrams daily of vitamin C had a 30 percent higher rate of respiratory problems than people getting more than 300 milligrams.

The study looked at wheezing and bronchitis, in particular. While it did establish an association between vitamin C intake and respiratory health, this kind of study can't tell us if vitamin C actually contributed to healthier lungs, says researcher Joel Schwartz, Ph.D., senior scientist at the Environmental Protection Agency. Vitamin C is involved in repairing oxidative damage in the lungs, however, and that may account for the findings, he says.

While Dr. Schwartz says it's much too early to make any recommendations, "certainly eating a little more broccoli isn't going to hurt you." One cup of cooked broccoli has 98 milligrams of vitamin C. (The U.S. Recommended Daily Allowance is 60 milligrams.) Other good sources include citrus fruit (124 milligrams per cup of orange juice), cantaloupe (67.5 milligrams per cup), strawberries (84.5 milligrams per cup) and green peppers (94.7 milligrams apiece).

High-sodium, low-potassium diets were also associated with more respiratory problems in the study, and increased fish intake was linked to fewer lung ailments.

STRONG-ARM TACTICS AGAINST DIABETES

Diabetics may someday have a strong incentive to lift weights: It may improve glucose tolerance, a study suggests.

Doctors have suspected for some time that aerobic exercise can improve glucose tolerance. But strength training is mostly uncharted territory. Researchers at the University of Maryland and Johns Hopkins University recruited 37 men and divided them into three groups. One group took up strength training, one took up jogging (an aerobic exercise), and one got no exercise. Blood tests were taken at the beginning and end of the 18-week study to assess glucose tolerance, the body's ability to metabolize sugar properly. That ability is impaired in diabetics. Both the strength-training and jogging groups saw significant improvements in glucose tolerance, with essentially no difference between them. The nonexercisers saw no changes. Both types of exercise lowered insulin levels, another positive change.

Participants in the study included prediabetics (glucose-impaired), Type II diabetics (non-insulin-dependent), and normal folk. Three of four prediabetic men who had strength training saw their glucose tolerance return to normal as a result. None of the diabetics returned to normal, "but they certainly improved," says one of the researchers, Ben F. Hurley, Ph.D., director of the exercise science lab at Maryland. He's currently checking out his theory that strength training has this effect because it increases muscle mass, which takes up some of the excess glucose from the bloodstream.

These results need to be replicated before anything is

certain, Dr. Hurley cautions. The improvements from strength training last at least 24 hours, he says, but whether strength training has long-term benefits that would warrant its use as therapy is unknown.

For now, he sees the possible value of strength training in the area of prevention. As people get older, their lean body mass tends to decrease, he notes. If older and diabetic people can retain or increase lean body mass through strength training, they may improve sugar metabolism.

The study also holds promise for people who aren't able to do aerobic activities. They may still be able to derive glucose-metabolism benefits from strength training.

If you have Type II diabetes, you might want to talk to your doctor about strength training. (There is no evidence that it is useful in Type I diabetes.)

LEAN-MEAT DIET RIVALS NO MEAT FOR HEART HEALTH

You can have your meat and heart health, too, a study from Australia confirms. Researchers there knew that vegetarians have lower blood pressure and blood cholesterol levels than people whose diets include meat. But meat eaters' diets generally include more fat.

So the researchers compared the effects of two diets with equal amounts of fat: one a vegetarian diet that included milk and eggs (lacto-ovo vegetarian), and another in which about half of the plant protein was replaced with lean meat. The effects of those diets were also compared to those of a typical high-fat diet.

Twenty-six men participated. Each spent six weeks on one of the diets, then six weeks on another.

Compared with the high-fat diet, both of the "prudent" diets significantly lowered blood pressure, total cholesterol, and low-density lipoprotein (LDL) cholesterol (the harmful kind). The vegetarian diet lowered cholesterol more than the lean-meat diet (a 10 percent versus a 5 percent decrease), but the drop in blood pressure was similar.

"Although the plant-protein–based prudent diet may confer the greater benefit, a more widely acceptable lean-meat–containing prudent diet appears to be almost as effective," the researchers say. "And a questionnaire answered by all subjects at the conclusion of the study showed a clear preference for the lean-meat prudent diet over both the high-fat and lacto-ovo vegetarian diets" (*American Journal of Clinical Nutrition*).

QUIT SMOKING AND RAISE HDL CHOLESTEROL

If you know someone who needs extra inducement to quit smoking, hit 'em with this: Within 30 days, they can halve the risk of heart disease caused by their low levels of beneficial cholesterol, according to one study.

Researchers at Florida State University found that high-density lipoprotein (HDL) cholesterol, the kind believed to help protect against heart disease, rose significantly in women who quit smoking. Eighteen women smokers began the study with an average HDL cholesterol reading of 50. After at least one month sans cigs, their HDL levels rose to an average of 60—comparable to those of nonsmokers. An increase of that magnitude is believed to reduce the risk of heart disease by two to three times, says Robert J. Moffatt, Ph.D., assistant professor of nutrition and movement science at Florida State.

VITAMIN C AIDS TREATMENT FOR ALLERGIC SKIN

Vitamin C supplements have been linked to improvement in the maddening skin problem known as atopic (allergic) dermatitis, preliminary research says. The problem is marked by redness, swelling, infection, and itching so intense that patients may be unable to sleep. It can be especially severe among children.

Researchers at the University of California at San Francisco studied ten patients with severe atopic dermatitis. The patients were between 3 and 21 years old. Each patient received either vitamin C or a placebo (blank pill) for three months. After a two-week "wash-out" period, the medications were switched. Neither the patients nor the researchers knew in which order the pills were given.

Both the severity and number of symptoms were reduced significantly while the patients were taking vitamin C. The number of infections was reduced, so that antibiotics were required only half as often. And there were no adverse reactions, according to study leader Glenn Kline, M.D., now associate clinical professor of pediatrics, University of Texas, Houston.

The vitamin C was given as an adjunct to standard therapy, which includes antihistamines (to relieve itching), oral antibiotics, topical steroids, and moisturizers. Dr. Kline sees the main value of the vitamin in this capacity. It is not a cure.

Dr. Kline decided to try vitamin C because the immune function deficits in people with atopic dermatitis are the same ones helped by vitamin C in other studies. The vitamin helps immune cells called neutrophils migrate toward infection sites, and helps change immune cells called lymphocytes from their small, resting stage to their large, active phase. These effects were noted in the study participants.

Dr. Kline cautions that patients shouldn't try this vitamin C regimen themselves. Consult a physician, he counsels, because people with kidney problems or a family history of such problems could encounter complications from large doses of vitamin C.

VITAMIN D DEFENDS AGAINST PSORIASIS

In the 1940s, doctors tried treating psoriasis with vitamin D. It didn't work. But now there's evidence that active vitamin D—the kind made by the kidney, not the kind found in supplements—may work.

The renewed interest in vitamin D started in 1984. Scientists discovered that exposure to active vitamin D inhibited the proliferation of skin cells and induced them to mature instead. That prompted the idea that active vitamin D may help treat disorders in which skin cells overmultiply—as happens in psoriasis.

The latest investigation of this theory comes from Osaka University Medical School, Japan. At random, 40 patients were given either one of two preparations of active vitamin D orally for six months, or a topical (rub-on) form of active vitamin D for eight weeks. All three treatments, especially the topical, significantly reduced psoriasis.

Furthermore, blood tests showed a significant relationship between the severity of psoriasis and the blood level of active vitamin D. The higher the vitamin D level before treatment, the less severe the psoriasis.

The Japanese study isn't conclusive. Still, vitamin D shows considerable promise as a safe and effective therapy for psoriasis, says Michael F. Holick, M.D., Ph.D., a vitamin D expert who pioneered the use of active vitamin D for psoriasis. In three to five years, he hopes to have Food and Drug Administration approval for treating psoriasis with vitamin D. In the meantime, you can keep up with the research by writing to Dr. Holick at the Vitamin D Laboratory, Boston University School of Medicine, Building M-1013, 80 E. Concord St., Boston, MA 02118.

Nutritional Healing Strategies

The Body Builders of Nutrition

Is your refrigerator an in-house pharmacy? Are doctors telling patients "Take two asparagus and call me in the morning"? Not quite. But these days there's more evidence than ever that good nutrition is good medicine. Nutritional factors play an important role in preventing cardiovascular disease and some forms of cancer. Careful meal planning can help control high blood pressure, elevated cholesterol, diabetes, and other conditions that you may think have nothing to do with nutrition.

With this in mind, here are 50 nutrition-for-health ideas. They range from the ready-to-use and scientifically verified to the over-the-horizon possible. The possibilities you should discuss with your doctor. The ready-to-use tips you can . . . well, use. Right now. Just keep in mind that nutritional medicine doesn't replace standard medicine but is an important part of it. And that if you have a serious illness, you should discuss any dietary therapy with your physician.

Remember, too, that none of these nutritional innovations changes the core principles of a healthful diet that have been recommended all along: Go low-fat, eat a variety of fresh fruits and vegetables, and substitute fish or fowl for red meat a few times a week.

Good nutrition won't cure everything, but it does have some preventive ways.

Abdominal Pain

Cookies calm tummyaches. This isn't permission for kids to pig out on Oreos. It's a serious remedy tested at the Children's Hospital of Eastern Ontario, in Ottawa. Researchers studied a group of 52 children who complained of recurrent stomachaches. Some of the children were given two high-fiber cookies, which are available in drugstores, per day. The rest were given two low-fiber cookies per day.

After six weeks, half the kids on the high-fiber cookies reported 50 percent fewer tummyaches. Only about one-fourth of the other kids reported that degree of relief from low-fiber cookies.

The researchers think that the children who seemed to benefit from "cookie therapy" needed more fiber in their diet to keep their bowels moving regularly. Slow-moving stools can cause constipation, sometimes triggering children's stomachaches. The researchers also point out that any chronic stomachache in children should be checked out by a doctor.

Arthritis

Fish oil is being tested as a possible treatment for rheumatoid arthritis. An Australian study published in the *Journal of Rheumatology* offers evidence that fish-oil capsules may bring relief to rheumatoid arthritis (RA) sufferers even when conventional forms of therapy have already been tried.

Twenty-three people undergoing long-term medical treatment for severe arthritis took 18 grams of fish oil daily for three months while a comparison group took a placebo (inactive substance). Results showed a reduction in joint soreness and also a measurable improvement in grip strength in the fish-oil group, but not in the placebo group. The researchers hypothesized that the fish oil worked by reducing levels of a substance (leukotriene B_4) known to cause inflammation. Because it isn't known whether long-term use of high doses of fish oil is safe, people with rheumatoid arthritis should consult with their doctor before trying this treatment.

Vitamin C May Help Bruising • Does Vitamin C curb bruising in RA? British researchers say that their preliminary findings suggest that correcting vitamin C deficiencies in people with rheumatoid arthritis may have a dramatic effect on stopping the cutaneous hemorrhaging (bruising) frequently associated with the disease. Rheumatoid arthritis robs the body of vitamin C directly, and drugs used to combat RA also tend to drain the body of the vitamin.

The result is that the blood doesn't clot properly and capillaries become weakened—preconditions for bruising. In their study (which has yet to be confirmed), the researchers found that three elderly patients deficient in vitamin C experienced dramatic and rapid improvement in their bruises when they took 500 milligrams of vitamin C daily. Doses of the vitamin, however, are unlikely to have the same effect on arthritis sufferers who are not vitamin C deficient.

Asthma

Doctors who treat asthma warn patients constantly against leaving home without their medication. But sometimes they just happen to do so. And that may be the time to reach for a nice hot pot of coffee, asthma experts say.

"Coffee contains naturally occurring chemicals quite similar to those that make drugs like theophylline effective asthma medications," explains Harold Nelson, M.D., senior staff physician for the National Jewish Center for Immunology and Respiratory Medicine. "In a pinch, drinking two or three cups of strong [regular] coffee has been reported to help control some asthma attacks.

"Unfortunately, several studies show absolutely no connection between coffee drinking and incidence of asthma," adds Dr. Nelson. So play it safe, say the experts:

Use your prescribed medications regularly and always have emergency supplies handy.

If you get caught without your asthma medication, by all means have a couple of cups—but start drinking before you start having trouble breathing. If you wait for an attack to begin, warns Dr. Nelson, the coffee may not have enough time to work.

Cancer

Several preliminary studies have linked low levels of vitamin D and higher risks of colon cancer. Normally, the body can manufacture vitamin D: the skin synthesizes it in the presence of sunlight. But some people living in the northern United States and Canada don't get enough sunlight in the winter months to manufacture adequate amounts of vitamin D.

Now another study has pointed to the association between vitamin D and less colon cancer. Researchers from Johns Hopkins University gathered blood samples from 25,620 volunteers in Washington County, Maryland. Over the next eight years, some of those people developed colon cancer. The researchers picked 34 of the colon cancer patients and matched each with two control subjects who did not get cancer but had similar profiles on certain key variables (for example, age, sex, race, and the month the blood sample was taken). After analyzing the respective blood samples, the researchers divided the volunteers into five groups based on vitamin D levels.

People with the lowest blood levels of vitamin D had four to five times the risk of getting colon cancer as those with the higher blood levels, according to study resuts published in the *Lancet*. Dramatic results from so small a sample need to be confirmed by other studies. And the possibility that calcium is working with vitamin D to reduce colon cancer risk needs to be studied. Still, it seems like a good idea for people above the Mason-Dixon line to make sure they get enough vitamin D from their diet during the colder months. Milk fortified with vitamin D is probably the most convenient source for both vitamin D and calcium.

Carotenoids, Vitamins C and E for Cervical Cancer •
Women who regularly consume vegetables rich in carotenoids (which the body converts into vitamin A) and fruit
juices rich in vitamin C may substantially reduce their risks
of cancer of the cervix, report researchers from the University of Washington. Their study of the dietary habits of
416 women found that women consuming the most dark
green and yellow vegetables had a 60 percent lower risk of
cervical cancer, while abundant intake of fruit juices was
associated with a 70 percent lesser risk. A high intake of
foods containing vitamin E was also linked to lower risk of
the disease.

Lowering Fats May Boost Cancer Protection • It seems that
reducing dietary fat may be a wise move for more than just
the heart and waistline.

A study by scientists from the University of Massachusetts Medical School, St. Luke's-Roosevelt Hospital
Center in New York, and other centers has found that
reducing dietary fat can enhance the activity of potentially
cancer-fighting natural killer (NK) cells. In men who lowered their fat intake, NK cell activity rose with each percent
decrease in fat consumed. The improvement was especially
significant in those men who ate more than 25 percent of
total calories from fat at the start of the study.

The results of the study support earlier animal and test-
tube studies suggesting that too much dietary fat may slow
the body's defenses against the cancer process "by depressing the tumor surveillance mechanisms of the immune system," the researchers said in their *American Journal of
Clinical Nutrition* report.

Vitamin A Derivatives Could Reverse Some Carcinomas •
Certain types of skin cancer have responded to experimental oral doses of vitamin A derivatives known as retinoids.
Basal-cell carcinoma has responded to both etretinate and
isotretinoin in a series of small studies involving 56 patients.
Approximately 50 percent of the cancer lesions showed
some response, with 9 percent clearing up completely.

Squamous-cell carcinoma has also been treated with retinoids. In several studies, a total of 14 patients with advanced cases of the cancer were given retinoids. Ten out of the 14 showed some positive response. Although the study samples are too small to prove whether retinoids are really effective, the results are promising.

As in the case of any other cancer treatment, retinoids should be taken under a physician's care. They're only available by prescription anyway. Pure vitamin A should never be used as a home substitute for retinoid therapy. It's just not the same, and it's toxic in large doses.

Allium Vegetables for Reduced Stomach Cancer • A preliminary study from China suggests that vegetables in the genus *Allium,* including onions and garlic, may reduce the risk of stomach cancer. The study, which was cosponsored by the National Cancer Institute (in the United States), surveyed the dietary habits of 564 stomach cancer patients and 1,131 randomly selected controls of similar sex and age. The patients and controls were all from an area of China with a high rate of stomach-cancer mortality.

The results: People who reported eating the greatest amount of onions, garlic, scallions, and Chinese chives had a significant reduction in their risk of stomach cancer. In fact, their risk was cut by more than half—down to 40 percent of the risk of people who rarely ate *Allium* vegetables.

Beta-Carotene Linked to Decrease in Oral Precancers • A study done in Arizona suggests that beta-carotene may reverse a precancerous condition called oral leukoplakia. Leukoplakia lesions can progress to full-blown cancer. They are common in long-term tobacco chewers and sometimes appear in smokers.

In the study, 25 patients were treated with 30 milligrams of beta-carotene per day. (That's the equivalent of eating about three to six carrots a day.) After six months of treatment, the lesions of 18 patients had decreased in size by 50 percent or more. (There were four complete remissions.)

Normally, only about 10 percent of patients with such lesions experience improvement without treatment.

Patients' skin might start turning yellow after a year on that dose of beta-carotene. The results, though, are quite promising. Beta-carotene is especially abundant in yellow-orange vegetables and fruits.

Fiber-Rich Foods May Protect against Colon Cancer • A number of population studies have found that people who eat a lot of fiber-rich foods have a lower incidence of colon cancer than those who don't get much fiber in their diet. The type of fiber associated with lower incidence? Insoluble fiber, which is found in vegetable stalks, potato and fruit peels, and the husks of whole grains.

Insoluble fiber isn't digested, and that may be the secret behind its protective effect. A large amount of insoluble fiber in the digestive system will help move feces through the colon quickly. Researchers think that may keep potential carcinogens (cancer-causing substances) from staying in contact with the colon for any length of time. But there may be other substances in high-fiber fruits and veggies that contribute to this possible cancer-shielding effect.

Raw Vegetables May Be Better Than Cooked • Diets rich in cruciferous vegetables, such as cabbage and broccoli, have been linked in studies to lower incidence of various digestive-system cancers. Some researchers speculate that any protective effect may be related to chemical compounds called indole glucosinolates that are present in these vegetables in significant quantities. But researchers from the University of Manitoba think that cooking makes glucosinolates break down into other, less-beneficial chemicals. Steaming and boiling may also be equally destructive to these cancer-fighting chemicals, although some do survive the process. So eating cauliflower and other cruciferous vegetables raw seems to be a prudent step.

Beta-Carotene Linked to Lower Lung Cancer Risks • A smoker's first move to reduce risks of lung cancer should be to quit. Another prudent step might be to eat more green and yellow vegetables rich in beta-carotene, a University of Minnesota study suggests. The blood levels of beta-carotene in smokers who had died of lung cancer were compared with those of smokers who were free of the disease. A significant difference was found between the two groups. The study provides "further evidence for a possible protective effect of beta-carotene against lung cancer among cigarette smokers," the researchers concluded in their report. Not just smokers may benefit from a diet rich in beta-carotene, however, as other studies have found a connection between beta-carotene intake and reduced risks of lung cancer in the population at large.

Dental Woes

Few foods are better for you than citrus fruits. But the word *citrus* refers to citric acid, and avid citrus drinkers could give their molars a potent acid bath. The solution is simple: "We recommend that people who are concerned about the effects of acidic juices on their teeth drink them through a straw," explains U.S. Department of Agriculture researcher Mike Faust, Ph.D. "That way, the juice doesn't even touch their teeth."

Cheeses May Offer "Secret" Protection • "Research suggests that certain cheeses—mostly the hard and aged Cheddar varieties—are beneficial to your teeth at the end of a meal," says Irwin D. Mandel, D.D.S. "But it's not because they neutralize acids. The plaque that forms on your teeth contains bacteria that emit their own acids. These acids leach calcium and phosphorus from your teeth. The calcium and phosphorus in cheeses like Cheddar may actually remineralize your teeth."

Key Nutrients May Halt Mouth Sores • A number of studies have found that about 15 percent of people who get canker sores are deficient in folate, iron, or B vitamins. Eating plenty of foods containing these nutrients or taking supplements in moderation can help eradicate the sores—but only if there was a deficiency to begin with. Chronic canker-sore sufferers who suspect a deficiency should check with their doctor.

Vitamin C May Speed Healing in Dental Surgery • A preliminary study from the University of Miami suggests that supplementing with vitamin C can shorten the healing time for tooth extractions. A total of 277 patients who took 500 to 1,000 milligrams of vitamin C daily for a week after an extraction healed faster and reported less pain on average than 175 patients who didn't take vitamin C. The supplemented patients were also five times less likely to suffer from dry socket (inflammation of the open socket), a common complication. Early results from a follow-up study using a placebo pill confirmed these initial findings. The researchers speculate that the vitamin might work by stimulating the immune system and scar-tissue formation.

Diabetes

Does bread made from whole wheat flour get digested the same as bread made from whole, unmilled wheat kernels? No, report Canadian researchers in the *British Medical Journal,* and that could be important news for people with diabetes. The researchers had diabetics eat breads that varied in their "whole flour" versus "whole grain" content. And they discovered that the greater the amount of whole, unmilled kernels in a bread, the more slowly the bread digests, and, therefore, the less it causes glucose (blood sugar) to rise. Avoiding such surges in glucose is crucial in controlling diabetes.

These results suggest the importance of "particle size," the researchers say. Even though a whole flour may contain all the essential parts of the wheat kernel, milling pulverizes these parts enough to substantially alter the speed with which they are digested. "Breads containing a high proportion of whole cereal grains may be useful in reducing the postprandial blood glucose profile [after-meal rise in blood sugar] . . . because they are more slowly digested," the researchers conclude.

High Fiber, High Carbohydrates Help Control Blood Sugar • Doctors used to recommend a high-protein diet and discouraged bread, potatoes, and other starches as well as fruits, vegetables, and simple sugars for diabetics. Today all that has changed.

Based on research over the past decade, the American Diabetes Association now advocates a high-fiber, complex-carbohydrate, low-sodium, low-fat diet. Research has found that fibers in whole grains, beans, and many fruits and vegetables help stabilize blood sugar.

A high-fiber, high-carbohydrate diet also helps peel off pounds, the only thing many Type II (non-insulin-dependent) diabetics have to do to eradicate or control their disease. Another benefit: Some research shows that diabetics with retinopathy (inflammation of the retina) eat diets significantly higher in protein and lower in fiber and carbohydrates than those without this condition. Finally, by choosing high-fiber foods instead of fatty foods, diabetics avoid putting themselves at risk for heart disease, the leading cause of death among diabetics.

Digestion Problems

Peppermint soothes tummy turbulence. After-dinner mints in restaurants can do more than sweeten your breath after a garlic-laden entrée. A strong peppermint candy mint or a mug of peppermint tea can help settle minor stomach discomfort. Oil of peppermint relaxes the muscle that closes the "door" from the esophagus to the stomach. This can allow excess gas to escape, relieving the feeling of over-fullness.

Not every candy mint works, though, because some of the more common brands contain artificial mint flavoring. But some better domestic and imported brands are made with true oil of peppermint. (Check the list of ingredients.) Most teas use peppermint leaves, which contain the oil. Of course, if you are prone to heartburn caused by a weakness in the esophageal opening, or if you find that peppermint is irritating, this remedy may be more trouble to your stomach than your original bellyache. Most adults have no problem, though. Peppermint tea should not be given to infants or young children because the menthol can cause a choking sensation.

Experimental Concoction May Offer Buffer against Turista • That seemingly invincible enemy of the exotic vacation, traveler's diarrhea, may finally have met its match. Scientists from the University of Maryland hope so, anyway. They've come up with a concoction made from cow's milk that, in an initial test, seemed to protect against the dreaded affliction. Since bacteria called *E. coli* are the most common cause of turista, the researchers decided to test the effects of a concentrate made from the milk of cows that had been immunized against the bacteria. And sure enough: Ten volunteers given the concentrate proved immune to a drink containing *E. coli*. The protection was not shared, however, by ten other people who had been given a concentrate made from the milk of cows that had been immunized against a bacteria other than *E. coli*.

How soon might the milk "cure" lead to a product available to consumers? All the researchers can say is that the results of their experiment are "highly encouraging," and further studies are under way.

Heart Disease

While fish-oil supplements get all the press, the health benefits of the original source of the oil should not be overlooked. Fish is a very lean alternative to red meat: 3 ounces of cooked Atlantic salmon (one of the fattiest fish) have less than one-third the total fat of 3 ounces of broiled rib-eye steak.

Not only is fish low in fat, but it's become common knowledge that the kind of fat it contains—omega-3 fatty acids, the working components of fish oil—is good for your heart. True, there's some controversy about the overall cholesterol-lowering properties of omega-3's. But researchers agree that omega-3's lower the liver's production of triglycerides, a particularly bad type of blood fat. Also, omega-3's seem to reduce the tendency of blood to form clots. (A likely scenario for a heart attack? A blood clot plugging a cholesterol-narrowed artery.)

For these heart-smart reasons (and perhaps some as yet undiscovered), try to eat fish two or three times a week.

Onions and Garlic May Fight Stray Blood Clots • Researchers are investigating the possibility that regularly eating fresh garlic and onions may protect against heart attack. Substances in the oil of these vegetables seem to inhibit the formation of blood clots (a principal trigger of most heart attacks) by making platelets less sticky. (Platelets, which circulate with red and white blood cells, are the prime clotting factor in blood.) This effect has been studied in test tubes, animals, and humans.

An occasional Mediterranean meal probably won't do very much. Regular use of onion and garlic (such as a side dish of cooked onions, raw onion in a salad or garlic in spaghetti sauce) would be most beneficial, according to Eric Block, Ph.D., chairman of the Chemistry Department at the State University of New York at Albany.

One warning: Some people may experience garlic and onion overkill. The stomach lining can become very sensitive to certain substances in these foods, causing gastric discomfort.

Other High-Fiber Foods Lower Cholesterol • By now you probably know that certain foods, such as oat bran and psyllium, which contain lots of water-soluble fiber, can effectively lower blood cholesterol. Less well known is the news that other high-fiber foods may be equally effective. Barley, carrots, apples, citrus fruits, and legumes (including dried peas, beans, and lentils) fall into this category. And animal studies suggest that rice bran, which contains only half the soluble fiber of oat bran, may also lower cholesterol as well as oat bran. The newest addition to this roster is soy fiber, although research is in the earliest stages. Soy fiber can be stirred into beverages or baked into breads, muffins, casseroles, and other dishes.

High Blood Pressure

Potassium may influence high blood pressure. There have been a number of studies linking low intake of potassium and increased incidence of high blood pressure. A small but impressive study from Temple University School of Medicine goes one step beyond these findings. Ten men with normal blood pressure were put on two experimental diets: one providing normal, the other low amounts of potassium. The men spent nine days on each diet. On the normal potassium diet, their blood pressures showed no significant change. But when on the low-potassium diet, their average arterial pressure (which takes into account both systolic and diastolic pressures) increased from an average of 90.9 to an average of 95. The men also retained more sodium and fluid, according to a report in the *New England Journal of Medicine*.

One of the researchers speculates that a low potassium intake may cause the sodium retention that, over time, raises blood pressure. These findings need to be confirmed by other studies, but they underscore the importance of eating potassium-rich fruits and vegetables (see "Good Sources of Key Nutrients" on page 40).

Impotence

Reducing dietary fat may boost potency. The same high-fat diet that can clog the arteries leading to a man's heart also affect the smaller vessels that lead to the penis. It's estimated that one out of every three men over the age of 40 will have potency problems at some point. And clogged arteries may be responsible for nearly half of those problems, says Harin Padma-Nathan, M.D., codirector of the Research Center for Sexual Function at the University of Southern California. He has diagnosed over 2,000 men with arterial impotence.

While surgery has been used to restore the blood flow, a low-fat diet may prove a more desirable cure. Dr. Padma-Nathan points out that an extremely low-fat, vegetarian,

Good Sources of Key Nutrients

- Vitamin A: Butternut squash, cantaloupe, carrots, collard greens, dandelion greens, pumpkin, spinach, sweet potatoes
- Vitamin B_6: Chicken, lentils, navy beans, red kidney beans, turkey breast, wheat germ (toasted)
- Vitamin C: Broccoli, brussels sprouts, cantaloupe, cauliflower, grapefruit, guava, kiwi, kohlrabi, mangoes, oranges, papayas, strawberries, tangerines
- Vitamin D: Cheese, milk, herring, mackerel, salmon
- Vitamin E: Almonds, margarine, mayonnaise, sunflower seeds, vegetable oil, wheat germ (toasted)
- Calcium: Almonds, cheese, figs, mackerel, milk, salmon, sardines, tofu
- Fiber (soluble and insoluble): Beans, blackberries, broccoli, brussels sprouts, corn, figs, legumes, oat bran, peas, prunes, raisins, raspberries, spinach, winter squash, wheat bran, whole grain breads
- Iron: Beans, fish, lean meats, nuts and seeds, poultry, tofu
- Magnesium: Almonds, cashews, corn germ (toasted), rice bran, sesame seeds, sunflower seeds
- Omega-3 fatty acids: Bluefish, herring, mackerel, salmon, trout, tuna
- Pectin (a form of soluble fiber): Apples, apricots, avocados, blueberries, carrots, figs, grapefruit, oranges, pumpkin, soybeans
- Zinc: Beef, peanuts, pork, potatoes, pumpkin seeds, turkey

low-stress prescription has helped reverse coronary artery blockage, so there's some reason to believe that whatever helps unblock one set of arteries could also help another. Even better: It's possible that men currently without problems may be able to prevent future impotence by carefully avoiding an artery-clogging diet to begin with.

Infections

A nutrient formula that fights infection? Doctors and nutritionists at the Shriners Burns Institute in Cincinnati,

Ohio, say that their preliminary research suggests that fish oil and other nutrients seem to boost their patients' immune system and reduce the likelihood of infection, a major complication in burn patients. About a third of 60 burn patients were put on the standard tube-feeding formula for burns; another two-thirds were put on a formula containing fish oil, extra zinc, and vitamins A and C. Those patients who were on the special formula recovered faster and had significantly fewer infections.

The researchers say that other studies need to be done before they're sure that their nutrient formula was really responsible for the patients' progress.

Vitamin E Linked to Tougher Immune System • Scientists know that vitamin E prevents oxidative damage to cells, improves white blood cell activity, and increases interleukin 2, a substance that promotes the growth of infection-fighting white cells called T-cells. It also turns off prostaglandin E, a naturally occurring substance that inhibits immune function.

And research appears to underscore vitamin E's importance to immunity. Jeffrey Blumberg, Ph.D., associate director of the U.S. Department of Agriculture's Human Nutrition Research Center on Aging, at Tufts University, gave 800 international units of vitamin E daily for 30 days to 16 healthy volunteers age 60 and over. Another 16 received a placebo. All the volunteers were put on a carefully balanced diet that included the U.S. Recommended Daily Allowance (USRDA) for vitamin E. When the researchers injected irritants under the skin of the volunteers, 80 percent of the group supplemented with vitamin E showed significant improvement in immune responses. Only 40 percent of people in the placebo group improved, while 40 percent worsened and 20 percent showed no change.

This study is not conclusive, but it does suggest the importance of incorporating whole grains, vegetable oils, and wheat germ in your diet to ensure adequate intake of vitamin E. Since the immune system begins to decline after puberty, getting enough vitamin E in your diet can benefit anyone over the age of 12.

Kidney Stones

Water dilutes stone-forming substances. Some people simply inherit the unfortunate tendency to develop kidney stones, but dietary habits also play a role. Kidney stones form when there is too much calcium in the urine. The calcium joins with oxalates or phosphates to form crystals that precipitate much the way salt crystals "snow" in water when you add more than the water can dissolve. One way to keep the crystals from forming is to dilute the crystal-forming particles in lots of liquid. The best way to do this? Drink lots of water. (Tea, however, is high in oxalates.) Many doctors recommend at least 2½ quarts daily.

Low Body Heat

A number of nonnutritional factors can foil the body's heating system (certain medications, Raynaud's disease, and dehydration, for example). But so, too, might a shortage of iron in the diet. It's believed that iron deficiency somehow alters thyroid metabolism, which is responsible for regulating body heat. Scientists from Pennsylvania State University got convincing evidence of iron's role in body heat when they asked women with iron-deficiency anemia and nonanemic women to sit in lawn chairs submerged to their necks in 82°F water. The anemic women wound up generating 13 percent less body heat than the nonanemic women.

Women, because they generally eat less, are more at risk than men for failing to get adequate iron in their diets. Among women between the ages of 15 and 44 the average consumption of iron is 10 to 11 milligrams per day, which is less than the Recommended Dietary Allowance (RDA) of 15 milligrams a day. To get your fair share of this mineral, look to foods like beans, lean meats, fish, and nuts and seeds. Before taking iron supplements, talk with your doctor.

Fish Oil Is Linked to Improvement in Raynaud's • Cold hands and feet a problem? The cause may be a circulatory disorder known as Raynaud's disease. And scientists have investigated the possibility that fish oil may help ease this problem by reducing the painful blood vessel spasms that cause a shutdown of blood flow to fingers and toes. In a preliminary study, researchers at Albany Medical College in New York found that symptoms of Raynaud's stopped completely in 5 out of 11 people who took fish-oil capsules daily for 12 weeks. The other 6 people were found to be able to extend by 50 percent the amount of time they could keep their hands submerged in cold water before experiencing a blood-flow shutdown.

The researchers caution, however, that these findings haven't yet been confirmed and that Raynaud's sufferers should not take fish oil without first checking with their doctors.

Migraines

It's now well established that certain edibles are capable of causing migraine headaches in some people. One headache trigger migraine sufferers should avoid is monosodium glutamate (MSG).

"MSG can be used anywhere, anytime, on almost any food," warns emergency medicine specialist George Schwartz, M.D. Sometimes a label reveals MSG's presence in a food product. But hydrolized vegetable protein (HVP), a flavor enhancer, may contain up to 20 percent monosodium glutamate. And labeling laws allow it to be identified simply as "flavoring" or even "natural flavoring." And kombu extract, a common ingredient in some health foods, is nothing more than MSG that's been extracted from seaweed.

Dr. Schwartz suggests that if you're MSG-sensitive and you're eating out, tell the waiter you don't want MSG or seasoning salt. He also recommends that you avoid processed soups, sauces, salad dressings, canned tuna, and cold cuts.

Motion Sickness

Ginger seems to have a quieting effect on traveler's nausea, according to researchers. Ginger ale has always been a home remedy for a mildly upset stomach. And powdered gingerroot worked better than Dramamine in widely quoted preliminary research from Brigham Young University.

In that study, 36 students who said they were highly susceptible to motion sickness were given either 100 milligrams of Dramamine, two capsules (940 milligrams) of powdered ginger, or two capsules of a neutral herb preparation. All the students were tested for nausea in a revolving chair (maximum test time: 6 minutes).

The group of students who took gingerroot were able to stay in the chair longer than either of the other groups without getting sick.

Powdered ginger capsules are commercially available in health food shops and some other stores. If you prefer to use your own spice rack, you can dissolve a quarter of a teaspoon of ginger in hot water or fruit juice.

Overweight

Fiber may help peel off pounds. A year-long study in Norway has added "bulk" to the growing evidence that dietary fiber can aid weight loss. Two diet plans were compared—calorie restriction plus a daily fiber supplement (taken in four individual doses 15 minutes before eating) and calorie restriction alone. After 27 weeks, the fiber group had lost an average of 8.4 pounds, while the nonfiber group had lost an average of 6.2. What's more, during a 25-week follow-up, the fiber group lost an additional 6.4 pounds despite being allowed to eat whatever they wanted. Perhaps the fiber curbed hunger, so the fiber group ate less, the researchers say (see "Good Sources of Key Nutrients" on page 40 for many excellent food sources of fiber).

Pectin May Thwart Overeating • Hollow legs take heart: A natural, water-soluble fiber called pectin may help put the brakes on runaway appetites. Researchers from the University of Southern California found that adding 15 grams of pectin (about half an ounce) to the meals of nine obese people increased the time required for food to exit their stomachs by an average of about 45 minutes. Such slowed-down digestion can dampen the appetite, partly by boosting feelings of fullness. While eating the pectin meals, the people decreased their food intake enough to lose an average of 6.6 pounds over a period of a month.

The researchers attribute pectin's digestion-slowing talents to its ability to increase the viscosity (thickness) of a meal as it gets processed by the stomach. A coauthor of the study, Jorge E. Valenzuela, M.D., says pectin may be of value in conjunction with other therapies to help curb certain disorders of overeating.

Hot Foods May Boost Calorie Burning • Those south-of-the-border spices may burn more than just your tongue—they may help "burn" calories, report researchers from Oxford Polytechnic in England. Hot spices may boost post-meal metabolic rate by as much as 25 percent, the scientists say. They offer as evidence their study of 12 people who were fed two 766-calorie meals that were identical except for their spice content. The one meal contained 3 grams of chili sauce and 3 grams of mustard sauce, while the other meal was left "cool." Result: Metabolic rates were raised more after the hot meal than after the cool one. The effect lasted more than 3 hours.

If this finding is real, it poses some interesting possibilities and questions. Can eating hot foods help you control your weight? Does the boost in metabolism accompany all foods that burn the tongue? To this latter question the researchers say no. Ginger, they say, seems not to fan the body's calorie-burning furnace.

Parkinson's Disease

Researchers are heartened by the possibility that physician-monitored megadoses of vitamins C and E may postpone the incapacitating symptoms of advanced Parkinson's disease. In a small study at Columbia University, 17 patients in the early stage of the disease were put on this experimental vitamin therapy. Compared to other patients, the group on vitamins was able to function 2½ years longer without drug treatment for advanced Parkinson's.

How might vitamins affect a mysterious nervous system disease like Parkinson's? Part of the answer may be found in free radicals—roaming molecular fragments (they're missing an electron) that are common in the body. When these fragments steal electrons from other molecules in the body, they damage tissue. They may play a role in parkinsonian nerve damage. Vitamins C and E are known antioxidants. They scoop up free radicals and neutralize them.

The researchers, of course, still need to verify these findings. People with Parkinson's interested in this study should not try this treatment on their own but should talk to their doctor about it.

Low-Protein Diet Assists Parkinson's Drug • Parkinson's patients become disabled because their brain doesn't produce enough dopamine, a natural chemical that allows the brain's motor system to work. Most patients can be helped by the drug L-dopa, which is changed into dopamine by the brain. L-dopa helps control the muscle tremors, rigidity, and slow movements that make daytime functioning difficult. To be effective, L-dopa must travel through the bloodstream to the brain using the same mechanism that transports amino acids. After a high-protein meal, amino-acid concentrations in the bloodstream can load up that transport mechanism and block out L-dopa, according to Jonathan H. Pincus, M.D., chairman of neurology at Georgetown University Medical Center.

So for patients who intermittently have symptoms of Parkinson's disease despite L-dopa therapy, Dr. Pincus and researchers at other centers are prescribing a restriction of daytime protein intake. On this program, patients eliminate most high-protein foods (meats, fish, eggs, legumes, and dairy products) from their breakfast and lunch menus. They compress most of their nutritionally required protein intake into an evening meal eaten shortly before bedtime. Amino acids flood the bloodstream for a few hours while the patient is asleep, blocking L-dopa when it matters least. This approach must be tried only under a doctor's care.

Pregnancy and Childbirth

Women who regularly take multiple vitamins around the time of conception may reduce by as much as 50 percent their risks of having babies with certain types of birth defect, report researchers from the Centers for Disease Control in Atlanta. A study of about 3,200 women found that, compared to nonmultivitamin takers or women who had been taking multivitamins only after conception, regular multivitamin takers experienced fewer births of babies with spina bifida (exposed spinal cord) or anencephaly (missing brain or skull bones). Regular vitamin intake was considered to be at least three times a week for three months before conception up through at least the first trimester.

"At this time, it is not possible to say whether this difference in risk is the direct result of vitamin use or the result of other characteristics of women who use multivitamins," say the researchers. "Further research is needed." They also caution that a woman anticipating becoming pregnant always should check first with her doctor before taking vitamins. The head of the study, Joseph Mulinare, M.D., also reminds women that there are other important steps they can take to prevent birth defects. These include not smoking, eliminating alcohol intake, using medications wisely, and getting prenatal care before becoming pregnant.

Magnesium May Help Moms-to-Be • In one study, Swedish researchers found that pregnant women who took magnesium supplements were less likely to hemorrhage, to have cervical problems, or to retain fluid than pregnant women who didn't get extra magnesium. The supplemented women's new babies were also more responsive and more likely to be of normal size than the newborns of the women not receiving magnesium. The researchers monitored 568 pregnant women from their third month of pregnancy through delivery. Half the women got 360 milligrams of supplemental magnesium per day. The other half got inactive pills.

These findings coincide with other research suggesting that magnesium deficiency in expectant mothers may result in serious complications. Studies done in this country show that most pregnant women get only about 160 to 260 milligrams of magnesium a day from food—considerably less than the Recommended Dietary Allowance (RDA) of 320 milligrams for pregnant women.

So moms-to-be should make a special effort to keep their magnesium intakes up to par, the experts say. Getting magnesium naturally in the diet is the best way. (Good sources include whole grains, leafy greens, nuts, and tofu.) Only after consultation with her doctor should a pregnant woman consider taking magnesium in supplemental form.

Vitamin A May Help Preemies Breathe • Scientists have suspected for some time that vitamin A is protective of lung tissue in adults, but now there is evidence that the vitamin also may help baby the lungs of premature infants. Doctors at Vanderbilt University Medical Center divided into two groups 40 premature infants suffering from inadequate lung development; one group received vitamin A injections every other day and the second received a placebo injection of salt water. After four weeks, the two groups were compared and some significant differences were seen. Only 9 of the 20 babies in the vitamin A group had gone on to develop a lung disorder common among premature babies known as bronchopulmonary dysplasia, while 17 of the 20 controls had developed the disorder. What's more, only 4 of the vitamin A babies remained in need of mechanical breathing assistance compared to 11 in the control group.

The need for supplemental oxygen and intensive care was less among the vitamin A babies, and they also suffered significantly less airway infection.

Respiratory Ills

Vitamin C may put a dent in the common cold. A study shows that, under controlled laboratory conditions, vitamin C may reduce the severity of cold symptoms. Elliot C. Dick, Ph.D., professor of preventive medicine and director of the respiratory-virus research laboratory at the University of Wisconsin, studied 16 men with nearly identical vitamin C levels. He gave half of them 500 milligrams of additional vitamin C four times a day and the other half a placebo. Then he locked the men in a dormitory for a week with eight other volunteers who had been deliberately infected with a cold virus. The 16 men continued their vitamin C or placebo treatment for two weeks afterward.

The results? Seven of the eight healthy men in the placebo group caught colds, while six of those taking vitamin C came down with colds. No significant difference here. But there was a big difference between the two groups in the severity of their colds. Dr. Dick explains that the men who didn't take vitamin C had symptoms twice as severe as the men who did take it. Compared to the vitamin C group, there were three times as many sneezes, twice as many coughs, and almost twice as many nose blows in the placebo group.

Spicy Foods May Help Relieve Congestion • Whether the congestion is due to bronchitis, asthma, allergies, or just a whopper of a cold, spicy foods may help clear the tracts. "Anything that adequately stimulates the stomach . . . will stimulate a reflex in the lungs that increases the production of a more mobile mucus, which is more readily expectorated," says Irwin Ziment, M.D., chief of medicine at Olive View Medical Center, an affiliate of UCLA School of Medicine. He has been studying the mucus-moving effects of spicy foods for years.

Best mucus-busters of all are horseradish, Tabasco, hot mustard, chili pepper, curry, and garlic, Dr. Ziment says. The amounts required for an effect are no greater than those typically found in Mexican or Indian foods, for example, eaten frequently.

And spicy foods are good for nasal and sinus congestion, too. As a rule of thumb, "If it makes your eyes water, it's going to make your nose run," Dr. Ziment says. People with gastrointestinal problems or a delicate stomach should check with their doctor before trying this remedy.

Skin Disorders

Can fish oil soothe psoriasis? Some early-stage research has at least raised the possibility of a nondrug treatment for this disorder. The study of 26 men and women suffering from psoriasis found that 58 percent of them got significant relief from redness, scaling, and skin plaques after taking 30 milliliters of fish oil daily for four months. Another 19 percent felt mild improvement.

Since there was no comparison group, the study could not prove whether fish oil was responsible for the improvements. Many experts believe that fish oil isn't highly effective alone, but may complement conventional drug therapy. Experts also caution against taking fish oil except under medical supervision, because long-term effects can increase the risk of the toxic effects of vitamins A and D. The best course of action for you to follow is to talk to your doctor about these preliminary findings before trying fish oil on your own.

Vitamin A Promotes Wound Healing • A review of numerous studies in the *Journal of the American Academy of Dermatology* confirms that vitamin A in the diet stimulates wound healing, especially in people who are taking steroid drugs. Steroids are often prescribed to control inflammation, but this also makes skin slower to heal. Vitamin A deficiency also slows wound repair. Since vitamin A is the most commonly deficient vitamin in the Western world, eating a vitamin A–rich diet may also speed healing of cuts or burns in many people who aren't taking steroids.

Severely injured patients, especially burn victims, often develop vitamin A deficiencies. All this is good reason to get enough vitamin A in your diet, especially if you've suffered from a wound or will be undergoing surgery.

Steroids suppress inflammation, while vitamin A tends to stimulate some aspects of inflammation in the presence of steroids. So consult a physician before taking more than the RDA of this nutrient.

Urinary Tract Infections

An old folk remedy may be gaining scientific backing. In research in both mice and humans, scientists found that cranberry juice seemed to prevent certain types of bacteria from clinging to the inside of the bladder and urinary tract. In one study, 15 out of 22 people showed this antiadherence effect in the urine 1 to 3 hours after drinking 15 ounces of cranberry cocktail. None of this proves that cranberry cocktail can stop a urinary tract infection. On the other hand, maybe Mom's old remedy is worth a try.

Vision Problems

Beta-carotene is linked to less eye disease. Regular consumption of fruits and vegetables rich in beta-carotene (for example, carrots, broccoli, spinach, and apricots) is associated with a lower risk of a leading cause of visual impairment known as macular degeneration (a degeneration of the retina), a study shows. The vitamin may exert a protective role by helping to reduce the harmful effects of exposure to ultraviolet light, University of Illinois researchers speculate. Their study, which examined the characteristics and eating habits of 3,000 people over 45, found that people who ate fruits and vegetables rich in beta-carotene on a daily basis had only about half the prevalence of macular degeneration as people whose intake of fruits and vegetables was extremely low.

Women's Health Problems

Calcium may be linked to fewer premenstrual woes. The results are preliminary but nonetheless encouraging. Researchers at New York Medical College tested calcium supplementation against a placebo in 33 women who suffered from premenstrual syndrome (PMS). The study followed the women for a period of six months. Women were given 1,000 milligrams of calcium carbonate or a placebo daily starting the first day of their periods for three months, then the regimens were switched: Calcium takers got placebos and vice versa for another three months.

The results: 72 percent of the women reported significant relief during the calcium-supplemented period. The women had less pain, water retention, and mood swings during ovulation, and they had less pain during menstruation. Only 15 percent of the women in the test reported relief while taking the placebo.

These findings still have to be checked by other research. In the meantime, the researchers say that women suffering from PMS should discuss calcium supplementation with their doctors.

Does Cutting Down on Salt Protect Bones? • Some physicians and nutritionists have long suspected that excess salt in the diet might weaken a woman's bones, since salt is thought to increase the amount of calcium leaving the body. Now a small study conducted in Canada lends some support to that suspicion, focusing on the group most at risk of low-calcium complications: postmenopausal women.

Researchers reporting in the *American Journal of Clinical Nutrition* fed 17 healthy postmenopausal women various amounts of salt. With an increase in salt intake, more lost calcium was detected in the women's urine. The researchers report that the amount of calcium the women got in their diet didn't seem to matter; whenever the women used extra salt, they lost significant amounts of calcium.

The researchers speculate that adding sodium, even within ranges normal in the American diet, may cause a healthy postmenopausal woman to lose as much as 10 percent of her total calcium stores over a ten-year period, putting her at risk for osteoporosis.

This connection between salt and calcium needs to be confirmed in larger studies. In the meantime, the low-sodium diet often recommended for general health is a prudent course.

Red Pepper, the Hot Healer

By Michael Castleman

The fiery taste and bright red appearance of red pepper (*Capsicum annuum* and *C. frutescens*) rank it among the world's most easily noticed spices. Recently the herb known variously as cayenne; capsicum; chili pepper; and Tabasco, Louisiana, African, and Mexican pepper has become as "hot" medically as it is on the tongue—in the field of chronic pain relief.

Red pepper has been a culinary staple in India and Asia for thousands of years. It was also used extensively in equatorial Africa long before Africans came in contact with white civilization. But the pungent herb was unknown in Europe until Columbus returned with it from his first voyage to the New World. The term "cayenne" comes from *kian*, its name among the Tupi Indians of northeast South America who gave the plant to Columbus. Today Cayenne is the capital of French Guiana. But ironically, South America exports only a tiny fraction of the millions of pounds of red pepper imported into North America each year. Most comes from India and Africa. (Peppers from Sierra Leone are reputed to be hottest.) Tabasco or Louisiana pepper grows along the Gulf Coast. Because so little red pepper comes from around Cayenne, the American Spice Trade Association considers the term *cayenne* a misnomer, and uses the more generic term *red pepper*.

"Violent Fruit"

After Columbus, European herbalists quickly incorporated red pepper into traditional herbal medicine. In his influential herbal (1652), Nicholas Culpepper, the London herbalist who castigated the university-trained physicians of his day for attempting to monopolize medicine, wrote that when used sparingly, "this violent fruit" was of "considerable service" to "help digestion, provoke urine, relieve toothache, preserve the teeth from rotteness, comfort

53

a cold stomach, expel the stone from the kidney, and take away dimness of sight."

Red pepper has long been used as a digestive aid in India, the East Indies, Central Africa, Mexico, and the Caribbean.

The first North American to use it medically was Samuel Thomson (1769–1843) of New Hampshire. From an early age, Thomson was fascinated by botany—and Indian botanical medicine. Although uneducated, he began calling himself "doctor" after successfully treating his family's and neighbors' ills with herbs. Thomson believed most diseases were caused by cold and cured by heat. He prescribed "warming" herbs extensively, chief among them red pepper. In 1813 Thomson patented a collection of herbal remedies (the forerunners of later "patent medicines") which he sold outside the channels of 19th-century mainstream medicine. At the height of its popularity in the late 1830s, Thomson's populist medicine claimed an estimated three million adherents. By 1850, Thomsonian medicine had fallen from fashion, but it helped spur the development of eclectic medicine, a more scientific—but still alternative—form of botanically oriented medicine, which flourished from the 1840s until the early 20th century and has since evolved into naturopathy.

The Eclectics' classic text, *King's American Dispensatory* (1898), recommends red pepper as a digestive stimulant, a treatment for colds, cough, and fever, and externally for muscle and joint stiffness (arthritis and rheumatism). The Eclectics also advised putting powdered red pepper in socks to treat chronic cold feet.

American folk healers have also recommended dusting children's hands with powdered red pepper to stop thumb-sucking and nail-biting.

Contemporary herbalists prescribe capsules of red pepper powder as a digestive aid, for colds, and bowel problems, and externally, for arthritis and rheumatism.

Pain Relief

For centuries, herbalists have recommended applying a paste made with red pepper to the skin to treat muscle and joint pains. Medically, this is known as a "counterirritant," a treatment that stimulates superficial inflammation to relieve deeper inflammation. Several counterirritant products containing red pepper are available over the counter, among them, Heet and InfraRub.

Recently, however, red pepper has been shown to possess true pain-relieving (analgesic) properties for one specific kind of chronic pain. For reasons not completely understood, capsaicin, the chemical that makes red pepper taste hot, renders the skin insensitive to pain by depleting "substance P," the chemical in the peripheral nerves that sends the pain message to the brain. Even where inflammation exists, without substance P, no pain message reaches the brain, hence there is no sensation of pain. Several studies have shown capsaicin to be so effective at relieving skin pain, a prescription analgesic cream containing the chemical has been licensed by the Food and Drug Administration under the brand name Zostrix.

Zostrix is the most effective treatment yet for "postherpetic neuralgia," severe, chronic pain following the disease known as shingles (herpes zoster). Shingles is an adult disease caused by the chicken pox virus, varicella, a member of the herpes family (but not herpes simplex, which causes genital herpes and cold sores). Varicella lies dormant in the body for decades, then for unknown reasons reappears in some people as shingles, causing a characteristic rash. In otherwise healthy adults, shingles clears up by itself within three weeks. But some people—usually the elderly or those with other illnesses—suffer the severe, chronic pain of postherpetic neuralgia. Now, thanks to red pepper, they don't have to suffer as much. Zostrix also shows promise as a treatment for postmastectomy pain, and the ankle and foot pain in diabetics known as "burning foot syndrome."

Science has also confirmed red pepper's traditional use as a digestive aid and gastrointestinal stimulant. The herb stimulates the secretion of both saliva and stomach acids. Saliva contains enzymes that initiate the breakdown of carbohydrate, and stomach secretions (gastric juices) further digest food.

Red pepper also helps reduce blood cholesterol levels and the tendency for blood to clot internally, both significant risk factors for heart attack, the nation's leading cause of death.

Safety

Red pepper may cause burning of the fingertips in those with sensitive skin, a condition dubbed "Hunan hand" because it was first identified in a man who prepared a Hunan Chinese recipe that called for chopping quite a few red peppers. He wound up in an emergency room with severe hand pain.

Red pepper does not wash off the hands easily. (Washing in vinegar removes it best.) Even with careful washing, the pungent herb may remain on the fingertips for hours and cause severe eye pain if contaminated fingers touch the eyes.

In cultures with bland cuisine, such as traditional American meat-and-potatoes cooking, people often believe that highly spiced foods damage the lining of the gastrointestinal system and contribute to ulcers. Not so, according to researchers who used a tiny video camera to examine subjects' stomach linings after both bland meals and meals liberally spiced with red pepper. They reported no difference in stomach condition and concluded, "Ingestion of highly spiced meals by normal individuals is not associated with [gastrointestinal] damage." However, the herb may cause gastrointestinal pain in those with ulcers or ulcerative colitis. Some people also report burning on bowel movement.

Dosage

In food, season to taste. For a digestive-aid tea, use $\frac{1}{4}$ to $\frac{1}{2}$ teaspoon per cup of boiling water. For external application, mix $\frac{1}{4}$ to $\frac{1}{2}$ teaspoon per cup of warm vegetable oil.

100 Power Foods

Don't eat this. Don't eat that. Is this what most of today's nutrition advice sounds like to you—all negative?

Fortunately, there's a world of foods that are good for you, that you should eat, and that also happen to taste divine. Here's our list of the foods that modern research smiles on for a whole lot of reasons.

What they have going for them (besides tastiness) are several nutritional factors that have been associated with lower risk of disease. Factors like dietary fiber, beta-carotene, calcium, and other health promoters. Like lower fat and fewer calories, two hallmarks of diets designed for sensible weight loss. The evidence linking some of the factors to lower risk is strong; the evidence for others just promising. But each food—nutritious in its own right—has several potential protection factors going for it. So prudence makes them all good bets. Which is not to say that you should limit your diet to this list. After all, variety is the cornerstone of a nutritionally complete diet. Nor can you assume that these foods can provide absolute protection from health problems. No diet can do that. The idea is simply that centering your meals around these foods may increase your odds of living a slimmer, healthier life.

The Top 100

Each of the following food groups includes a list of healing factors, which apply to all or some of the foods in that group. See "Key to Health-Protecting Powers" on page 64 for a more complete description of the benefits.

Fish • You can't go wrong by including fish in your diet. Most fish are high in magnesium, potassium, phosphorus, zinc, and the B vitamins. Fish is also a good source of iron—in a form that's easier to absorb than iron from plant sources. **1. Flounder** (under 12 percent of calories from fat) and **2. haddock** (under 8 percent) are some of the trimmest fish in the ocean. But fattier fish are not all bad. In fact, the omega-3 fatty acids found in **3. tuna, 4. bluefish, 5. mackerel, 6. trout, 7. herring,** and **8. salmon** are what make them such smart choices.

- Blood fortification
- Heart health
- Normal blood pressure
- Weight loss

Poultry • Some of the best sources of iron on earth can be found flying above earth. Both **9. duck** and **10. goose** are high in the most absorbable type of iron. Goose is also rich in vitamin E.

For nearly as much absorbable iron, but much less fat, try **11. turkey** and **12. chicken.** With turkey, dark meat's the most iron-rich part. With chicken, breast meat is best.

- Blood fortification
- Cancer prevention
- Heart health
- Weight loss

Red Meats • While it's always been promoted as a good source of iron, red meat usually doesn't spring to mind when thinking about weight loss or heart health. Yet cuts of **13. extra-lean pork, 14. extra-lean beef,** and **15. extra-lean lamb** can qualify for these two benefits. Pork tenderloin, for example, gets only 26 percent of its calories from fat. When buying beef, look for the new "select" grade to get the least amount of fat. Trim all visible fat off even the best cuts before cooking. **16. Venison** is low in both fat and cholesterol.

- Blood fortification
- Heart health
- Weight loss

Shellfish • Certain shellfish could vie for the title of "Nature's Mineral Depository." At least three types are low in fat and rich in various minerals. **17. Clams** are so high in iron, it's a wonder they don't rust! Two dozen steamers provide over 150 percent of the U.S. Recommended Daily Allowance (USRDA), which is 18 milligrams per day. **18. Mussels** deserve recognition, in part because they are such an inexpensive source of nutrition. **19. Oysters** are iron-rich, too—but ounce for ounce, the Atlantic-bred variety is about 25 percent richer in iron than Pacific-grown species.

- Blood fortification
- Heart health
- Weight loss

Dairy Foods • There are no better natural sources of calcium than milk and other dairy products. But the fat content of regular milk may sabotage its health benefits for dieters. Enter **20. skim milk,** with only 2 percent of its calories from fat, and **21. 1 percent low-fat milk (solids added),** with 20 percent of its calories from fat. In addition, virtually all milk is enriched with vitamin D, which enhances calcium absorption. Add to your low-fat calcium source list **22. 1 percent low-fat cottage cheese,** any other **23. low-fat cheese,** and **24. nonfat yogurt.**

- Bone health
- Cancer prevention
- Heart health
- Normal blood pressure
- Weight loss

Cruciferous Vegetables • This nutrient-rich family of foods has been linked to lower incidence of colorectal cancer. Many of these vegetables are high in insoluble fiber, vitamin C, and folate. Major members of this family include **25. cabbage, 26. bok choy (Chinese cabbage),** and **27. cauliflower.**

    28. Brussels sprouts and **29. broccoli** sport a lot of calcium and iron, for a plant source, and beta-carotene. The iron and calcium aren't quite as easily absorbed as from animal sources, but some of it is absorbed nonetheless.

- Blood fortification
- Bone health
- Cancer prevention
- Heart health
- Normal blood pressure
- Weight loss

Orange-Yellow Fruits and Vegetables • 30. Winter squash, 31. cantaloupe, 32. apricots (especially dried), 33. mangoes, and 34. papaya are all rich in beta-carotene. **35. Carrots** are, ounce for ounce, one of the best sources of beta-carotene.

In addition to high beta-carotene levels, **36. sweet potato, 37. acorn squash, 38. butternut squash,** and **39. pumpkin** are all good vegetable sources of iron.

- Blood fortification
- Cancer prevention
- Heart health
- Normal blood pressure
- Weight loss

Dark Green Leafy Vegetables • 40. Romaine lettuce, 41. chicory, 42. endive, 43. watercress, 44. spinach, 45. kale, 46. Swiss chard, 47. arugula, 48. dandelion, and **49. turnip greens** are high in beta-carotene and vitamin C. Their dark green color is the clue.

Iron and calcium lurk in some greens, but the body can't make use of the minerals in these vegetables as efficiently as those from meats and dairy foods.

- Cancer prevention
- Heart health
- Normal blood pressure
- Weight loss

High-Carbohydrate Vegetables • No "empty starches" here! **50. Potatoes** are a nutritionist's dream: high in vitamin C, B$_6$, copper, magnesium, phosphorus, potassium, iron, and fiber.

51. Corn is no empty husk, either. It contributes vitamin B$_6$, folate, and fiber. And there's excitement about preliminary studies that indicate a possible cholesterol-lowering effect of corn bran.

- Blood fortification
- Cancer prevention
- Heart health
- Normal blood pressure
- Weight loss

Grains • Fiber and a wide variety of trace minerals (including iron) are the main health benefits in most grains. **52. Whole wheat pasta, 53. buckwheat, 54. barley, 55. wheat germ,** and **56. brown rice** are excellent examples. **57. Oatmeal** and related foods have been shown to lower cholesterol.

Most grains aren't very high in calcium. But **58. amaranth,** a little-known, highly nutritious grain, is an exception. (It can be boiled and eaten like rice, or ground into flour and used in hundreds of recipes.) **59. High-fiber cereal** and **60. whole grain bread** are usually fortified with calcium, iron, and a variety of vitamins.

- Blood fortification
- Bone health
- Cancer prevention
- Heart health
- Normal blood pressure
- Weight loss

Beans • Soluble fiber is the prime healing ingredient of this group. *Prevention* adviser James W. Anderson, M.D., advocates a diet high in beans (or legumes) for cholesterol control. In small studies, Dr. Anderson has seen cholesterol levels drop 60 points (in three weeks!) after adding **61. pinto beans** and **62. navy beans** to the diets of men with high cholesterol. All legumes, including **63. lima beans, 64. lentils, 65. kidney beans, 66. peas, 67. chick-peas (garbanzo beans),** and tiny **68. adzuki beans,** are high in iron and other minerals. **69. Anasazi beans** have a special attraction: all the nutrition of regular beans, but less than 25 percent of the flatulence-causing sugars.

- Blood fortification
- Heart health
- Normal blood pressure
- Weight loss

High-C Fruits • The prime advantage for these fruits is their high vitamin C content. Most are also good sources of potassium. **70. Kiwi** is no longer a stranger to most people. One kiwi packs almost 125 percent of the USRDA of vitamin C, which is 60 milligrams. **71. Acerola,** a West Indian fruit, still is a stranger. It looks something like a cherry, tastes very tart, and just one contains 134 percent of the USRDA. Welcome, stranger! **72. Pineapple, 73. honeydew melon, 74. pomegranate,** and **75. persimmon** are old high-C friends.

- Cancer prevention
- Heart health
- Normal blood pressure
- Weight loss

Citrus Fruits • A day without an **76. orange** is like a day without 116 percent of the USRDA of vitamin C. Citrus fruits are probably the best-known source of C. Most of us don't realize that they're also loaded with fiber (especially pectin, suspected of lowering cholesterol) in the stringy sections and inner peel. In fact, the original pectin versus cholesterol studies were done with concentrated fiber from **77. grapefruit.** The pink variety has a small amount of beta-carotene. **78. Tangerines** also contain some beta-carotene. And while few people will actually eat a **79. lemon** or **80. lime,** fresh-squeezed juice—over fish, or in sparkling mineral water as a low-cal lemonade—is a good source of vitamin C.

- Cancer prevention
- Heart health
- Normal blood pressure
- Weight loss

Peppers • 81. Sweet or bell peppers are superior vegetable sources of vitamin C. One cup contains 158 percent of the USRDA. Eat them raw, as a side dish. **82. Chili peppers** might be too spicy for some people's side dishes, but they're worth the heat: Just ¼ cup packs over 150 percent of the USRDA.

- Cancer prevention
- Heart health
- Normal blood pressure
- Weight loss

Berries • 83. Blueberries and other bite-size fruits are very high in vitamin C, fiber, and a few trace minerals. There's a superdose of fiber in the seeds of **84. raspberries** and **85. blackberries.**

- Cancer prevention
- Heart health
- Normal blood pressure
- Weight loss

Nuts and Seeds • Most nuts and seeds are very oily but packed with trace minerals. **86. Dried sunflower seeds** get 78 percent of their calories from fat, but they're an incredibly compact source of calcium, copper, iron, magnesium, phosphorus, potassium, zinc, and vitamin E. **87. Dried pumpkin or squash seeds** are comparable.

- Blood fortification
- Bone health

Dried Fruits • When dried, these fruits become concentrated storehouses for fiber and a variety of minerals, in-

Key to Health-Protecting Powers

Blood Fortification

Foods rich in iron, important for protection against anemia.

Bone Health

Foods rich in calcium, important for strong bones and teeth.

Cancer Prevention

Foods high in one or more of the following: insoluble fiber (associated with reduced gastrointestinal cancer risk), calcium (ditto), beta-carotene, folate (possibly able to halt cancerous progression in precancerous growths), vitamins C and E (linked in some unconfirmed studies to reduced risks). In general, a diet low in fat and high in fruit and vegetables has been linked to lower risk of cancer. Beta-carotene consumption has been linked in several studies with reduced cancer risks. One population study from the State University of New York at Buffalo, for example, compared the diets of 450 lung-cancer patients to those of over 900 healthy people. The results were strongest in men: Those with the lowest beta-carotene intake were 80 percent more likely to get lung cancer than those with the highest. The difference between high and low carotene intakes? The equivalent of one carrot per day!

Heart Health

Foods that are low in overall fat, high in the types of fat that seem to prevent artery clogging, high in vitamin C (thought to possibly change the ratio of "good" to "bad" cholesterol), and/or high in soluble fiber (thought to lower cholesterol).

Oat bran, which is packed with lots of soluble fiber, has so far been the best of the fiber cholesterol-busters. A study from the University of California,

(continued)

Key to Health-Protecting Powers—
Continued

Irvine, for instance, tested the effect of two oat-bran muffins per day on the cholesterol levels of 19 medical students. After four weeks, they had an average 5.3 percent reduction in total cholesterol and an 8.7 percent reduction in artery-clogging low-density lipoprotein (LDL) cholesterol. Control groups eating wheat bran or mixed wheat-and-oat muffins showed no such cholesterol reduction

Omega-3 fatty acids, found mostly in certain fish, lower blood fats called triglycerides and may reduce the risk of blood clots that could lead to heart attacks or strokes.

Normal Blood Pressure

Foods high in potassium, magnesium, and/or calcium. All are linked to blood pressure control. Calcium is used to lower blood pressure in some people with hypertension. Fruits and vegetables are high in magnesium and potassium.

Weight Loss

Foods that are low in fat, high in important nutrients, and moderately to very low in calories. Low fat is significant in weight loss because dietary fat is more easily converted to body fat than either protein or carbohydrate. Foods indicated with this benefit get no more than 30 percent of their calories from fat, which is the recommended benchmark for a healthful diet.

cluding copper, iron, magnesium, phosphorus, potassium and zinc. The fruits are low in fat, but high in calories. **88. Raisins, 89. dried peaches, 90. prunes,** and **91. figs** are *Prevention*'s dried fruit picks.

- Blood fortification
- Cancer prevention
- Heart health
- Normal blood pressure

High-Fiber Fruits • Some fruits, such as **92. apples, 93. bananas,** and **94. pears**, are fiber rich in their undried form. Much of the fiber in these fruits is pectin. Ten **95. cherries** provide 1 gram of fiber, much of it soluble.

• Cancer prevention
• Heart health
• Normal blood pressure
• Weight loss

Garlic Group • A few researchers suspect that **96. garlic** and related bulb vegetables may have a cholesterol-lowering effect. And don't forget **97. onions** and **98. leeks**.

• Heart health
• Weight loss

Oils • Kudos for **99. olive oil** and **100. canola oil** for their apparent cholesterol-fighting power. They contain large proportions of monounsaturated fats, which studies say may not only lower cholesterol but raise beneficial high-density lipoprotein (HDL) cholesterol.

• Heart health

Probiotics: New Evidence on a Culture That Cures

You know that dairy products provide a healthy dose of calcium. But a tantalizing trail of research suggests that two particular dairy foods—yogurt and acidophilus milk—may offer benefits that go beyond good nutrition.

What makes these milk products unique? Both contain live cultures of beneficial bacteria. Just 1 ounce of yogurt or acidophilus milk has several hundred million active microorganisms, estimates Frank E. McDonough, Ph.D., a food researcher with the U.S. Department of Agriculture.

These organisms initiate the fermentation process that transforms plain milk to tart-tasting yogurt. And, some experts suggest, they may protect the body in some astounding ways, possibly curing gastrointestinal problems, lowering blood cholesterol, and even helping to prevent cancer.

For years, some doctors have prescribed yogurt for patients taking antibiotics. That's because antibiotics have a nasty habit of loosening up our bowels while wiping out our infections. And yogurt has long been used to fend off diarrhea. Now there is scientific evidence to support its use.

To understand how yogurt goes to work, picture your intestines as a microcosm of organisms, some beneficial and some potentially dangerous. Fortunately, under normal conditions, good bacteria outnumber the bad by about 99 to 1. But when you take antibiotics, this ratio shifts in favor of the bad bugs.

"Antibiotics are designed to kill bacteria. Unfortunately, the good bacteria happen to be more susceptible to antibiotics than the bad," says Dr. McDonough.

Enter probiotics. While antibiotics indiscriminately kill the good bacteria with the bad, probiotics promote the good bacteria. "Probiotics means positively influencing the ratio of good to bad bacteria in your intestines," explains *Prevention* editorial adviser Manfred Kroger, Ph.D., a food science professor at the Pennsylvania State University who is researching and writing on the subject of probiotics.

For at least 40 years, scientists have been studying probiotics in test tubes and laboratory animals. Now, researchers at the University of Lille, in France, and Tufts University School of Medicine report the first controlled experiments on human beings.

At the University of Lille, ten volunteers took two 3-day treatments with the antibiotic erythromycin, chosen because of its reputation for causing diarrhea. During each treatment, the subjects also ate yogurt three times a day. For one antibiotic treatment, the yogurt contained live cultures of beneficial bacteria. But during the other, the yogurt had been heated to kill off all the bacteria.

The researchers discovered that only one of the subjects who ate the yogurt with active cultures developed diarrhea while taking antibiotics. But eight of the ten volunteers eating the heated yogurt developed diarrhea.

What's more, stool tests showed almost no clostridium bugs—the usual culprit behind antibiotic-induced diarrhea—in people eating the live yogurt cultures. But seven out of ten persons eating bacteria-free yogurt did have clostridium in their stools (*Lancet*).

Help for Colitis

Meanwhile, researchers at Tufts University School of Medicine are testing the use of acidophilus milk in people with recurrent colitis, an inflammatory condition of the large intestine that causes diarrhea.

Their study began with five people who had developed repeated attacks of colitis that were related to treatment with the antibiotics cephalexin, erythromycin, clindamycin, ampicillin, and penicillin. The subjects had suffered between two and five relapses of colitis, despite treatments with a variety of drugs. Each showed dangerous levels of clostridium bacteria in their stools during tests at the beginning of the study.

Each day the subjects took a concentrated dose of acidophilus bacteria in a teaspoon of skim milk. Within ten days, four of the five colitis sufferers had complete relief from their diarrhea, and minuscule or no amounts of clostridium in their stools. One subject needed a second treatment, which completely cured her symptoms. None of the subjects has had any further relapses of colitis. Colitis tends to recur in 10 to 15 percent of all cases of antibiotic-related diarrhea (*Lancet*).

Since these results were published, the Tufts researchers have repeated their study with 15 additional subjects and had the same encouraging results. Tufts researcher Sherwood L. Gorbach, M.D., says their findings suggest that acidophilus bacteria (such as the type found in cultured milk products) may help people with antibiotics-associated colitis by killing off stubborn clostridium bugs once and for all.

The Cancer Connection

In 1984, Dr. Gorbach and his colleague Barry R. Goldin, Ph.D., caused a stir in the scientific community by reporting evidence of a possible link between acidophilus and prevention of colon cancer.

The search for a "cancer connection" began with a very puzzling clue. A 1975 study showed that people in Finland do not have the same high rate of colon cancer that other inhabitants of the West suffer. And yet they eat the high-fat, low-fiber diet typical of Western societies.

"That led some of us to wonder whether the low colon cancer rate in Finns had anything to do with the huge amount of yogurt they eat—more per person than any other country in the world," says D. R. Rao, Ph.D., of Alabama A&M University.

Based on that discovery, Dr. Rao tested the protective effect of yogurt bacteria against cancer in laboratory rats. He was unable to establish a link with colon cancer, although he did note some success in preventing a type of ear tumor that does not appear in humans.

Later, however, Dr. Gorbach and Dr. Goldin at Tufts reported they had used acidophilus to stop bad bacteria in human colons from making enzymes that, at least in test-tube studies, produce compounds such as nitrosamines. Nitrosamines are one of the most feared cancer-causing substances, according to Dr. Kroger.

In the Tufts study, 21 men and women, average age 28, drank two glasses of plain milk every day for one month. After a four-week break, they spent another month drinking two glasses of milk containing acidophilus bacteria. Weekly stool samples tested during each period showed a 200 to 400 percent reduction in dangerous colon enzymes while the subjects drank acidophilus-spiked milk. Plain milk had no effect.

As promising as this sounds, Dr. Goldin says it's too early to say that acidophilus bacteria can actually prevent colon cancer. "We know now that acidophilus bacteria can somehow stop colon bacteria from producing certain enzymes. And we know that these colon enzymes will turn certain compounds into nitrosamines in the test tube," he says. "But it will take a lot more research to find out if what happens in the test tube happens in human beings— and whether eating foods with acidophilus actually leads to a reduction in colon cancer risk."

Next Target: Cholesterol

Meanwhile, probiotics researchers are busy looking into another lead—that is, to see whether cultured milk might reduce elevated blood cholesterol, a major risk factor in heart disease.

Fifteen years ago, a report noted that members of the Masai tribe of Africa have low cholesterol despite the fact that they eat a high-fat diet, which usually raises blood cholesterol. Like the Finns, the Masai are heavy consumers of cultured milk products. Unfortunately, further research on the possible cholesterol-lowering effect of cultured milk has yielded mixed results.

"I've had some very puzzling results," says Tufts researcher Dr. Gorbach. "I have tried to lower cholesterol levels with yogurt in about 150 people. Sometimes cholesterol went down, and sometimes nothing happened. I have no idea why yogurt worked sometimes and not others," he adds, "but I just know there's something there."

Stanley E. Gilliland, Ph.D., a scientist at the Oklahoma Agricultural Experimental Station, believes that some probiotics researchers have been stymied because they didn't use the right strain of cultured milk bacteria in their studies. In test-tube experiments, he's shown that some strains of acidophilus bacteria gobble up cholesterol, particularly in the presence of bile (digestive juices) and the absence of oxygen. "The same conditions exist in our small intestine," says Dr. Gilliland.

Dr. Gilliland also tested his acidophilus strain on pigs fed a high-cholesterol diet. Blood cholesterol levels in the acidophilus-treated pigs stayed down despite their cholesterol-rich diet. Meanwhile, blood cholesterol shot up in another group of pigs fed the same high-cholesterol diet, but not the special acidophilus bacteria (*USDA Animal Science Research Report*).

What to Look For in the Dairy Case

Finding yogurt is easy; your supermarket is bound to carry at least a half-dozen varieties. But be sure the yogurt you choose contains live cultures. If it doesn't, the label will say "contains no live active cultures." Also, be sure to look for low-fat or nonfat yogurts so you don't add unnecessary fat calories to your diet.

Some yogurts contain acidophilus bacteria in addition to the normal yogurt bacteria cultures. These will state "made with live acidophilus cultures" on the label.

Acidophilus milk is widely available in supermarkets. Although you might expect it to be sour, it's not. In fact, it's called sweet acidophilus milk because it's not fermented, as yogurt is. You can buy sweet acidophilus milk with 1 percent fat and use it in place of regular milk. It tastes the same. By the way, kefir, a low-fat yogurt drink, also contains beneficial bacteria.

The Oklahoma researcher now plans to study whether a selective strain of acidophilus can cut cholesterol in people with dangerously high blood levels. Since these bacteria work in pigs—and pigs and people have amazingly similar digestive and blood systems—there's a good chance that they could work in humans too, says Dr. Gilliland.

Meanwhile, what should we do while we await the outcome of current probiotics research?

"Even if it turns out that none of the claims is valid, and we continue to eat cultured milk products, we haven't hurt ourselves," says Dr. McDonough. "We get 85 percent of our calcium from dairy products like yogurt and acidophilus milk. And milk protein ranks second only to eggs—even before meat—as the highest-quality protein. So the beneficial effect is very high regardless of the outcome of current research.

"On the other hand, I'm convinced that there's enough evidence to show that the added benefits of cultured milk products are there," he says.

And cultured milk products are easier to digest—even for people with lactose intolerance. "Still, some people have a degree of difficulty digesting milk products, even cultured ones," explains Dr. McDonough. "Certainly, for them, a gallon a day would be too much. A cup of yogurt or acidophilus milk a day is reasonable."

Dr. Kroger agrees that a one-, two-, or three-cup-a-day approach is appropriate for most of us. "Cultured milk products are a good way to keep our digestive system in peak condition, and that will affect many other aspects of our health. Yogurt and acidophilus milk may be for the gut what jogging is for the cardiovascular system."

Echinacea: A Flower with Power

By Michael Castleman

Echinacea is the best-kept secret among medicinal herbs native to the United States. No other plant is so potentially important to self-care and mainstream medicine. And yet since the 1930s, echinacea's many benefits have been enjoyed almost entirely by Europeans. Fortunately, the situation is changing rapidly as echinacea regains its former prominence on this side of the Atlantic.

Echinacea (*Echinacea purpurea* and *E. angustifolia*) is native to the American Midwest and Plains and to South Central Canada. Known variously as purple coneflower, black sampson, and rudbeckia, most of the half-dozen species of this attractive four-foot perennial have purple daisylike flowers whose rays radiate from a cone-shaped center, hence the name purple coneflower. Once the rays fall, the central cone appears black, hence the black in black sampson. The sampson refers to the name Sampson, which was common among black slaves. Slaveholders saw a resemblance between echinacea's black flower cones and the heads of their slaves.

Early naturalists sent hundreds of North American plants, including echinacea, back to European universities for botanical classification. The man who classified echinacea was none other than Carolus Linnaeus (1707–1778), the Swedish botanist considered the father of modern scientific nomenclature. Linnaeus named the herb *Rudbeckia purpurea*, in honor of his botanical mentor at the University of Uppsala, Professor Rudbeck. *Purpurea* is Latin for "purple." The plant is still widely known as rudbeckia in Europe. Later botanists adopted the more descriptive name echinacea, based on the Greek term *echinos,* meaning "sea urchin," a reference to the spiny appearance of the flower's central cone. *Angustifolia* is a combination of two Greek words, *angustus,* "narrow," and *folium,* "leaf."

Indian Medicine

Echinacea was the Plains Indians' primary medicine. Root poultices were applied to wounds, insect bites and stings, and snakebites. Other tribes used the plant to treat colds, coughs, rabies, smallpox, measles, mumps, and muscle and joint pains (arthritis and rheumatism).

Plains settlers adopted the Indians' uses for echinacea, but the plant remained a folk remedy until around 1870, when a Nebraska physician, Dr. H. C. F. Meyer of Pawnee City, began using black sampson root both externally and internally to treat snakebite, particularly the bite of the venomous rattlesnake. It worked so well that Dr. Meyer developed an echinacea-based patent medicine called Meyer's Blood Purifier, which he claimed treated everything from eczema to syphilis.

Fifteen years passed, and in 1885, Dr. Meyer apparently decided it was time to share black sampson's amazing properties with his medical colleagues. He sent the plant—along with a glowing description of its many actions—to John Uri Lloyd, a professor at the Eclectic Medical Institute in Cincinnati, an alternative medical school operated by the 19th-century Eclectic physicians, who favored botanical medicines over bleeding and the mineral medicines (arsenic and mercury) routinely used by the orthodox physicians of

the time. The Eclectics were forerunners of today's natu-
ropaths, and at the time, the Eclectic Medical Institute was
one of the nation's leading centers of botanical research.
Lloyd identified Meyer's plant as *Echinacea purpurea* but
dismissed his claims as nonsense.

Undaunted, Dr. Meyer shipped some echinacea root to
Lloyd's Eclectic colleague, John King, who had mentioned
the plant's use by the Plains Indians in the first edition of
his Eclectic medical text, *King's American Dispensatory*
(1852). King was more receptive, and after successfully
using the herb to treat bee stings, chronic nasal congestion,
leg ulcers, and infant diarrhea (cholera), he extolled the
plant in an 1887 article in the *Eclectic Medical Journal* and
recommended it in subsequent editions of his *Dispensatory*.

By the publication of the 1898 edition of *King's American Dispensatory,* coeditor John Uri Lloyd had renounced
his earlier skepticism and declared the herb an effective
treatment for wounds, venomous bites and stings, blood
poisoning (septicemia), diphtheria, meningitis, measles,
chicken pox, malaria, scarlet fever, influenza, syphilis, gangrene, and even certain cancers. Lloyd's enthusiasm was
not simply academic. He was also a cofounder of Lloyd
Brothers Pharmacists of Cincinnati, the major formulator
of Eclectic medicines. Lloyd Brothers developed several
echinacea products, which enjoyed tremendous popularity
around North America as infection treatments from the
1890s well into the 1930s—despite denunciations in the
Journal of the American Medical Association, which called
the plant useless. During the 1920s, it was a rare medicine
chest that did not contain tincture of echinacea. But by the
1930s, as antibiotics became widely available, echinacea
fell from pharmaceutical favor. It was largely forgotten in
the United States until the herb revival of the 1970s.

Healing Properties

Fortunately, Europeans never discarded echinacea,
and old Dr. Meyer would be tickled to learn how therapeutic
the plant actually is. Many European (mostly German) studies since the 1950s have shown echinacea to have significant

antiviral, antibacterial, antifungal, and antiprotozoan properties, thus lending credence to its traditional uses in wound
healing and treatment of the common cold, flu, and many
other acute infectious diseases.

The herb's antimicrobial action is due in part to the
presence of chemicals called echinacosides; echinacea also
exerts an additional antimicrobial effect by strengthening
cell membranes against assault by invading microorganisms. Cell membranes contain a gel-like chemical called
hyaluronic acid (HA), which acts as a shield against microbial attack. To enter cells, many pathogens produce the
enzyme hyaluronidase, which dissolves HA, allowing them
to penetrate cell membranes and cause infection. But echinacea contains the chemical echinacein, which counteracts
hyaluronidase, thus preserving cells' HA coating, and preventing infection.

Echinacea further inhibits infection by exerting a powerful immune-stimulating effect. Once infected, cells secrete
chemicals that attract infection-fighting white blood cells
called macrophages to the area. Macrophages (literally,
"big eaters") engulf and destroy the microbial invaders. A
1984 study showed echinacea boosts the macrophages' ability to destroy pathogens.

Echinacea also fights infection through an effect similar
to that of the body's own virus-inhibiting chemical, inter-
feron. Before a virus-infected cell dies, it secretes inter-
feron, which boosts the ability of surrounding cells to resist
viral assault. Echinacea does essentially the same thing. In
one study, researchers bathed cells in echinacea root extract, then exposed them to two virulent viruses, influenza
and herpes. Their rate of infection was 50 to 80 percent
below that of untreated control cells. These findings have
led even herbal medicine critics to write that echinacea
"may result in . . . clear improvement in such conditions
as the common cold."

Tests of echinacea in people have produced equally
dramatic results. In a 1986 German study, 203 women with
recurrent vaginal yeast infections caused by the fungus *Candida albicans* were treated with either an antifungal cream,

or the cream plus echinacea. The echinacea group received the herb either by injection or by mouth. After six months, 60 percent of the women treated with just the antifungal cream had experienced recurrences, but among those also treated with echinacea, the figure was only 16 percent, a highly significant difference. The women in the echinacea-injection group showed greater initial benefit than those who'd taken the herb orally, but after ten weeks, all differences disappeared, demonstrating the effectiveness of taking the herb by mouth.

This study's positive result led researchers to wonder if the echinacea had exerted a direct anti-*Candida* effect, or a more general immune-boosting response. Using classic skin scratch allergy tests, they checked the echinacea group's reactions to the bacteria that cause tetanus, diphtheria, and tuberculosis. The larger the skin welt preduced, the greater the immune system reaction to the microbe. Compared with controls, those taking the echinacea produced much larger welts, suggesting that the herb's effectiveness against yeast infection was simply a small part of a more generalized immune-enhancing action.

Echinacein, the chemical that prevents microbial invaders from secreting the enzyme that breaks down the cells' hyaluronic acid coating, also spurs wound healing. Wounds covered with a salve containing echinacein knit faster, apparently because the herb's HA-protective effect increases the productivity of skin-forming cells. This finding confirms echinacea's original use in wound treatment.

HA also helps lubricate the joints. Joint inflammation (arthritis) breaks down HA, but echinacea's HA-protective action exerts an anti-inflammatory effect, thus lending credence to the herb's traditional use as a treatment for arthritis.

Finally, a 1972 study showed that echinacea contains a substance that is active against lymphocytic leukemia, raising the possibility that the herb may one day be used to treat cancer.

In Germany, where botanical medication is more mainstream than it is in the United States, echinacea is widely used externally to treat wounds and internally to treat colds, influenza, bacterial and fungal infections, and herpes sores. The Germans even have an echinacea toothpaste with reported periodontal benefits.

Safety and Dosage

The Food and Drug Administration (FDA) lists echinacea as an herb of "undefined safety," but the medical literature contains no reports of adverse effects. So echinacea can be considered safe in usual doses for otherwise healthy, nonpregnant adults. However, there have been reports of bulk echinacea being adulterated by other herbs. Any adulteration would reduce the herb's effectiveness, and depending on the adulterant, might cause adverse reactions. Fortunately, several U.S. herb companies market prepackaged echinacea powder and tincture under FDA purity guidelines.

If you buy packaged echinacea, follow the package directions. If you buy the herb in bulk, mix 2 teaspoons of powdered root per cup of water, boil, than simmer 15 minutes. Drink up to three cups a day. Using tincture, take a teaspoon up to three times a day. Echinacea tastes sweet initially, then bitter, and often produces a tingling sensation on the tongue.

Your Healthy Heart

Good News on Clearing Coronary Blockages

The bad news first: Big problems remain or are being newly discovered with virtually all of the promising mechanical technologies of the past decade designed to clear blocked blood vessels.

Lasers, balloons, "shavers," you name it. Yes, they do a great job of clearing the accumulation of a lifetime's worth of American living out of your arteries. But it comes back. Sometimes worse than it was before.

Now the good news: Three different studies show that you can slow down—even reverse—blockages without surgery. Two used a combination of drugs and high doses of niacin. The other used no drugs at all.

Study #1: Colestipol and Niacin

From the University of Southern California School of Medicine: a study of 103 men who all had previously undergone coronary bypass surgery. Half were put on drug therapy: colestipol (which prevents cholesterol from being absorbed by the body) plus high-dose niacin; half got look-alike placebos with no real drug or niacin.

They've now been followed for four years. Actual angiograms (pictures of the inside of their blood vessels) show that the progression of existing blockage has been slower by about half in those who got the real drugs. More impressive, only 12.5 percent of the guys getting the real drug therapy developed new blockages as compared to 38.3 percent of those getting the placebos.

But this therapy was *not* benign. The high doses of niacin caused lots of hot flashes and dry, itchy skin. The colestipol caused a "significant" number of gastrointestinal complaints.

In one man, the colestipol caused gastrointestinal bleeding so severe that he required surgery.

Study #2: Add a Different Drug, Use Less Niacin

At the University of Washington, Seattle: a study of 105 men with bad low-density lipoprotein (LDL) cholesterol levels, family history of heart disease, *and* active symptoms of heart trouble.

They were divided into three groups: One got dietary counseling alone. One took niacin and colestipol. One took colestipol and lovastatin, a less intense cholesterol attacker. All got angiograms. If the blockage got worse by 10 percent, the disease had "progressed." If it got better by at least 10 percent, it was regressing. Obviously, this is one time when the men didn't want to progress.

Regression occurred in 10 percent of the "diet only" group. But 45 percent of them got worse.

In the two drug groups, however, an average of 35 percent got better and only 23 percent got worse.

More important: The number of bypass operations, angioplasties, and heart attacks was reduced by 75 percent in the groups that got the drugs.

The researchers say that by using lower doses of the niacin and drugs, they virtually eliminated the side effects.

Study #3: No Drugs at All

From the Preventive Medicine Research Institute, Sausalito, California: Beginning four years ago, researchers took 48 men whose angiograms showed substantial blockages (but who, for one reason or another, decided not to have surgery) and gave them a choice.

They could gently modify their lifestyle (no more than 30 percent of calories from fat, moderate exercise, and try to stop smoking) or they could begin a new life: no animal products except for skim milk, egg whites, and nonfat yogurt. No oils. No more than 10 percent of calories from fat. An hour of stress-reduction techniques a day (meditation, yoga, or stretching). An hour of exercise three times a week. If they smoked, they quit.

Half made the easy changes; half took on the new life. Only one dropped out.

In the "new life" group, the average percentage of vessel blockage has gone from 41.4 percent down to 37.8 percent. In the group that tried moderate changes, it's gone up from an average of 44.1 percent to 46.2 percent.

Coronary flow—the amount of blood getting to the heart—increased measurably in the new lifers. It got worse in the others. Perhaps most important, symptoms such as angina virtually disappeared in those who radically changed their lifestyle.

Two things have been proven, say the researchers. One is that the system works; at the end of a year results are as good or better than any drug therapy.

The other is that people can and will stick to it.

Cut Your Cholesterol: A New and Simple Plan

Mirror, mirror on the wall, What risks heart disease most of all—high blood pressure or high cholesterol, lack of exercise or too much stress, Type A behavior or a fatty diet, family history or cigarettes?

If scientists had the answer, heart disease might not still be our number one killer. In fact, heart disease comes at us from many directions. Researchers do know this—

and feel free to post it on your refrigerator door—lowering high serum cholesterol (above 200) lowers risk.

Some controversy has cropped up in the news regarding this dictum. But it can be reported confidently that the stir was little more than a flash looking for a pan. Virtually every major health organization in the country immediately responded with outrage that the importance of cholesterol should even be questioned, much less debunked. From the National Heart, Lung and Blood Institute, for example, came the remark that what needs to be discussed is not whether high cholesterol levels need to be reduced but rather how they should be reduced.

Cholesterol counts, and a lot. Researchers have been able to calculate that a person's risk of heart disease drops by 2 percent every time his or her cholesterol level drops by just 1 percent. If that fails to impress you, try doing some quick arithmetic. If Fred lowers his cholesterol from 265 to just under 200—a drop of 25 percent—he has cut his risk of heart disease in half. The information in this chapter may help those of you who can achieve a substantial reduction in your serum cholesterol level, easily and safely, through dietary changes alone.

What sort of changes? The game plan is a wonderfully simple one: Eat more of the foods that can help lower cholesterol and less of the ones that can raise it. It's a one-two punch that could, if your cholesterol level is currently high, reduce your risk of heart disease by as much as 50 percent.

Step #1: Go for Soluble Fiber

Fiber comes in two basic styles—insoluble, found in wheat bran and the indigestible parts of vegetables and fruit; and soluble, prevalent in oat bran, oatmeal, citrus fruits, and most types of beans. As for the difference between the two types, it's quite simple: Insoluble fiber does not dissolve in water, which makes it great for promoting regularity (and reducing risks of colon cancer), while soluble fiber does dissolve in water, which makes it great for cleaning out cholesterol.

How? Maybe by flushing cholesterol out of the small intestine before it has a chance to get to artery walls. Some scientists theorize that soluble fiber binds with bile, a digestive fluid that contains goodly amounts of cholesterol, in a way that causes the bile to be excreted in the stool. The result: less cholesterol circulating in the bloodstream, where it can cause trouble.

Research by *Prevention* adviser James W. Anderson, M.D., shows that the addition of soluble fiber to the diet can have a significant and immediate impact on high cholesterol levels. In one study, Dr. Anderson found that men with cholesterol levels around 260 experienced 60-point drops in just three weeks (*American Journal of Clinical Nutrition*). In another, longer study, cholesterol levels averaging 294 fell by 76 points in six months. That's a 26 percent reduction! And it didn't take truckloads of soluble fiber to achieve these impressive results. The amount in a mere 1½ cups of beans daily, or a single cup of oat bran daily, did the trick. Other very preliminary research suggests that the soluble fiber in rice bran and apple pectin may share these same cholesterol-dissolving powers. Include a tasty variety of all of these cholesterol-bashers in your diet, and your cholesterol could suddenly find itself without a leg to stand on.

Step #2: Take a "CSI" Tally

Of course, the best cholesterol-lowering diet is also one that's light in saturated fat and cholesterol—which brings us to the second (and easier) part of our plan. Easy because it means no more confusion over just how heart healthy, or heart hazardous any given food actually is. Is lobster, for example, which is high in cholesterol but low in saturated fat, a better or worse choice than a broiled steak, which is lower in cholesterol but high in saturated fat? Is a piece of pizza worse for the arteries than a hot dog? "CSI" to the rescue.

CSI stands for Cholesterol/Saturated-Fat Index, a formula that correctly weighs the effects of both a food's cholesterol and its saturated fat on blood cholesterol. Scientists have known for some time that both food constituents have a cholesterol-raising effect, but not until the CSI formula (developed by registered dietitian Sonja L. Connor, and William E. Connor, M.D., of Oregon Health Sciences University) was there a way of computing their combined effects. The formula works as follows: A food's saturated-fat content, measured in grams, is multiplied by 1.01, while its cholesterol content, measured in milligrams, is multiplied by 0.05. The two products are then added to yield the food's CSI rating.

What this shows is that both the cholesterol and saturated fat you eat are important. They both interfere with the liver's ability to remove cholesterol from the bloodstream. It's something to keep in mind as you read through the CSI table on page 84.

How to Use the Table

Remember, the higher a food's CSI rating, the greater its tendency to raise levels of cholesterol in the blood—and hence your risk of heart disease. For optimum cholesterol-lowering results, your goal should be to eat foods totaling a CSI of no more than about 28 a day if you're a moderately active woman, and no more than about 36 a day if you're a moderately active man. (These figures assume daily calorie intakes of approximately 2,000 and 2,800 respectively, and are based on a diet deriving approximately 25 percent of its calories from fat.) Feel free to achieve lower daily CSI numbers for greater cholesterol reduction. (For a complete copy of the CSI, send $5 to OHSU-L465, Heart Publications, 3181 SW Sam Jackson Park Rd., Portland, OR 97201. For additional information on the CSI, consult the Connors' book, *The New American Diet System,* published by Simon & Schuster.)

THE CHOLESTEROL/SATURATED-FAT INDEX

Food/Portion	CSI	Calories
Breakfast Dishes		
Pancakes, three 4″		
Regular	8	258
Modified (made with oil, skim milk, no yolks)	1	212
French toast, 1 slice		
Regular	5	131
Modified (made with skim milk, egg substitute)	<1	116
Omelet		
Plain, 2 eggs	27	244
With cheese, 2 eggs	34	350
Egg whites only, ½ cup	0	48
Egg substitute, ½ cup	2	127
Cereals and Grains		
Bran flakes, 1 cup	0	127
Granola, 1 cup		
Commercial with soy oil	3	495
Commercial with coconut oil	17	503
Cooked cereal, 1 cup		
Wheat	Trace	126
Oat bran	Trace	103
Oatmeal	Trace	145
Rice, 1 cup		
White	Trace	223
Brown	Trace	179
Breads and Tortillas		
White, whole wheat, raisin, rye, or pumpernickel bread, 1 slice	Trace	70
Pita pocket	Trace	180
Crescent roll	3	101
Corn tortilla		
Baked	Trace	52
Fried	1	63
Cheeses		
Cottage cheese, 1% fat, ½ cup	<1	81
Swiss, 1 oz.	6	107
Cheddar, Monterey Jack, Colby, Havarti, longhorn, 1 oz.	8	114
Part-skim ricotta, 2 Tbsp.	2	39
Cream cheese, 1 oz.		
Regular	8	99
Reduced-fat	5	74
Dairy Products		
Milk, 1 cup		
Whole	7	149

Food/Portion	CSI	Calories
1% fat	2	102
Skim or powdered nonfat	1	85
Cocoa with skim milk, sugar-free, 1 cup	2	68
Yogurt, 1 cup		
Plain	7	141
Low-fat, plain	3	143
Nonfat, plain	<1	127
Sour cream, ½ cup		
20% fat	18	234
Light, 10% fat	10	180
Half-and-half, 1 Tbsp.	1.5	20
Nondairy creamer, 1 Tbsp.		
Powdered	2	33
Liquid	<1	20
Milkshakes, 16 oz.		
Soda fountain	32	671
McDonald's	5	304
Appetizers		
Guacamole, ¼ cup	1	62
Sour-cream dip, ¼ cup	8	111
Liver pâté, 2 Tbsp.	7	72
Soup, 1 cup		
Minestrone	1	83
Split pea, lentil	2	170
Swedish meatballs, 3	12	287
Pizza and Pasta		
Pizza, thin crust, 2 slices		
Cheese	16	552
Green pepper, mushroom, onion	9	419
Pasta, 1 cup	Trace	192
Egg noodles, 1 cup	3	200
Spaghetti with meat sauce, 1½ cups	6	356
Ravioli, cheese, with tomato sauce, 6 large or 12 small	10	216
Poultry (boneless, cooked)		
Chicken, Cornish game hen or turkey, white meat, 3 oz.		
With skin	6	178
Without skin	4	140
Ground chicken or turkey, 3 oz.	5	154
Frankfurter, 1	5	102
Giblets, 3 oz.	18	135
Liver, 3 oz.	28	133
Fish and Shellfish (cooked)		
Salmon, canned, ½ cup	3	138
Tuna, canned (water packed), ½ cup	2	102

(continued)

THE CHOLESTEROL/SATURATED-FAT
INDEX—*Continued*

Food/Portion	CSI	Calories
Fish and Shellfish (cooked)—continued		
Trout, rainbow, 3 oz.	4	115
Sea scallops, 8	2	90
Clams, steamers, 25 medium	3	81
Shrimp, ⅔ cup	9	99
Lobster, 1½ tails	3	101
Meat (boneless, cooked)		
Beef, 3 oz.		
Corned beef, pastrami	15	316
Short ribs	15	323
Sirloin tip	9	215
Tenderloin, porterhouse	15	323
Flank	5	161
Ground beef, 3 oz.		
20% fat	11	246
15% fat	9	215
10% fat	7	170
Venison, 3 oz.	5	168
Lamb, 3 oz.		
Stew meat, lean	7	189
Chop, shoulder	17	323
Leg	10	219
Liver, 3 oz.	22	161
Pork		
Tenderloin, 3 oz.	5	141
Sausage, 4 links	12	295
Spareribs, 3 oz.	13	309
Beans (cooked, no fat added)		
Navy, pinto, kidney, black, ½ cup	Trace	106
Lentils, split peas, ½ cup	Trace	115
Tofu (bean curd), ½ cup	<1	79
Fruits and Vegetables		
Apple, pear, peach, 1 medium	Trace	60
Melon, berries, 1 cup	Trace	60
Canned fruit, ½ cup	Trace	60
Coconut, raw, ½ cup	12	142
Carrots, celery, green beans, tomatoes, broccoli, cauliflower, raw, 1 cup	Trace	25
Peas, corn, potatoes, winter squash, ½ cup	Trace	65
Salads		
Green salad, 1 cup		
No dressing	Trace	10
With blue-cheese dressing, 2 Tbsp.	3	147
With French dressing, 2 Tbsp.	3	140
With Italian dressing, 2 Tbsp.	1	97

Food/Portion	CSI	Calories
Potato salad, 1 cup		
German-style	2	163
With mayonnaise	10	392
Tabbouleh, 1 cup	3	269
Three-bean salad, 1 cup	4	287
Fats and Spreads		
Butter, 1 tsp.	3	36
Margarine, 1 tsp.		
Stick	1	35
Diet	0.3	17
Liquid	<1	35
Mayonnaise, 1 Tbsp.		
Regular	2.1	101
Light	0.8	51
Oils		
Canola, safflower, corn, olive, 1 tsp.	0.5	41
Palm, 1 tsp.	2	41
Coconut, 1 tsp.	4	41
Frozen Desserts		
Frozen yogurt, low-fat, 1 cup	3	144
Sherbet, 1 cup	3	270
Ice milk, soft-serve, 1 cup	4	224
Ice cream, 1 cup		
10% fat	15	269
12% fat	19	349
18% fat	30	684
Popsicle, 1	0	99
Fudgesicle, 1	Trace	91
Baked Goods		
Cinnamon roll	5	276
Danish pastry	8	235
Doughnut		
Plain	4	153
Frosted, with coconut	7	309
Carrot cake, one 3″ square	14	662
White cake from mix with water, egg whites (cocoa frosting), one 3″ square	3	319
Cheesecake, one slice	22	355
Cookies, 2		
Oatmeal	4	186
Chocolate-chip	18	186

SOURCE: Adapted from *The New American Diet System,* by Sonja L. Connor, M.S., R.D., and William E. Connor, M.D. (New York: Simon & Schuster, 1991).

Nibble Your Cholesterol Down

There's more good news on the cholesterol front: It's not just what you eat but how you eat that can help lower your heart disease risk. Small meals eaten frequently appear to be better for keeping cholesterol levels in check than large meals eaten infrequently. How so?

In an article published in the *New England Journal of Medicine,* researchers from the University of Toronto explain: Large meals appear to cause the release of large amounts of insulin. That in turn seems to stimulate the production of an enzyme that increases cholesterol production by the liver. High insulin levels also are suspected of harming arteries directly by stimulating the laying down of both fat and muscle cells on the inside of artery walls. The result can be a thickening effect, which may help lay the foundation for the kind of arterial blockage of which heart attacks are made.

Small meals, however, appear to avoid these undesirable effects. The University of Toronto study found that both insulin and cholesterol levels decreased significantly when test subjects ate their normal number of daily calories in numerous small meals throughout the day rather than their usual three squares. In just two weeks, insulin levels dropped by 28 percent and total cholesterol fell by an average of 8.5 percent. What's more, low-density lipoprotein (LDL) cholesterol (the so-called bad kind) was reduced by 13.5 percent. Granted, the people in the study were obliged to eat every hour on the hour to achieve these reductions, for a total of 17 meals daily, but as the study's director, David Jenkins, M.D., Ph.D., says, "We believe that this model illustrates an important principle. . . . Increasing meal frequency while maintaining constant caloric intake may have a role in the prevention of heart disease."

The Truth about Oat Bran

"Oat bran debunked!" scream the newspaper head-lines; "Oat bran found *not* to lower cholesterol levels," shout the evening news reporters.

Horse hockey (as old Colonel Sherman Potter on "M*A*S*H" would have said)! It's a shame that so many people who report the news can't take the time to read the actual study instead of a news release.

Researchers Ensured Failure

Oat bran had about as much chance of looking good in this study as you do of winning money from a street-corner game of three-card monte.

It's safe to assume that many of the people who have turned to oat bran in an attempt to improve their health in recent years are those at increased risk of a heart attack—mostly men, mostly older, all with high cholesterol levels. (Otherwise, why would you care about bringing it down?)

It makes sense, therefore, that that's who you'd test, right? Like the classic studies that originally showed oat bran to be effective.

Not the Boston researchers whose work so grabbed the headlines. They tested only 20 people. Sixteen of them were women. The average age was 30.

Did they *at least* have high cholesterol levels to begin with?

No. The average cholesterol levels at the beginning of this study were *so* low that you could add 25 points and they'd still be in the desirable range!

But the Deck Was Stacked Even More

These young, healthy women with low cholesterol lev-els (mostly dietitians, by the way, who revealed at the end of this "double-blind" study that they knew all along just when they were taking the oat bran) went on a low-fat diet. For six weeks they ate 100 grams of oat bran daily. For another six weeks they ate "a low-fiber refined wheat prod-uct" (Cream of Wheat).

However, although the diets were *supposed* to match each other exactly, the researchers admit that "the high-fiber foods contained approximately 3 grams more fat than the low-fiber versions"—some of which came from oil that was presumably considered necessary to prepare the oat-based foods, but not the wheat.

The end result was that every day for six weeks, the people taking the oat bran got *more* total fat, *more* saturated fat, *more* polyunsaturated fat, *more* monounsaturated fat—or simply put, *more* of every type of fat known.

Even the researchers had to admit that "dietary fat was significantly higher during the oat-bran period than during the wheat period."

Even with a Stacked Deck, Oat Bran Worked!

Giving oat bran to young women with low cholesterol levels is a lot like pouring water into the empty gas tank of a car. Okay, the car still won't move, but then again—why did you think it would?

But even with this scientific equivalent of Mike Tyson defending his title against Mother Theresa, oat bran's potential to improve cholesterol levels somehow managed to squeeze through.

You won't find it in the summary (known as an "abstract") that precedes the article. You won't find it in the conclusions. But sift through the raw data and you'll see that, compared to when they ate the Cream of Wheat, the oat bran raised these people's high-density lipoprotein (HDL) cholesterol levels (the "good" kind) and lowered their low-density lipoprotein (LDL) cholesterol levels (the "bad" kind). And that's *despite* the extra fat they were fed.

Trust the Old Studies Instead

Journal of the American Dietetic Association, June 1986: 208 people, half men, half women, *without reducing their fat intake,* lowered their total cholesterol by around 6 percent by adding between 35 and 39 grams (about 1½ ounces) of oat bran a day to their diets.

The *American Journal of Clinical Nutrition,* December

1984: 20 men with high cholesterol levels, most with some form of heart disease, lowered their total cholesterol by 19 percent (around 40 to 50 points) by eating either 100 grams of oat bran or 119 grams of beans a day. Both foods worked equally well.

At least three other studies—all testing people much more appropriate than those tested in the "new" one—got similar results: Oat bran will lower cholesterol when given half of a fair chance to do so.

We're *not* saying that oat bran is a cure-all. Obviously, a low-fat diet *has* to be the first step in any cholesterol-lowering program. And other high-fiber foods, such as beans, may work just as well as oat bran in lowering cholesterol when added to such a diet.

The point is that you don't test a handful of young, healthy women who work in your hospital—who have no reason to lower their already "desirable" cholesterol levels—stack the deck with added fat, and then go screaming from the rooftops that oat bran is a failure.

All the evidence indicates that high-fiber foods are beneficial when added to the diet of the people who actually *need* them—the people at risk for heart disease. The people who want to work to avoid a heart attack.

So please don't stop eating high-fiber foods such as oat bran because of this "study." It's already done enough damage.

Countdown to Lower Blood Pressure

If you thought that drugs—with their unwanted side effects—were the only way to control high blood pressure, think again. Studies show that a sizable number of people with mild hypertension can get their pressure dropped *without* drugs.

At an American College of Cardiology meeting, two

separate studies reported that nondrug therapy achieved control equal to drugs for people with mildly elevated blood pressure. In some cases, the nondrug techniques worked even *better* than drugs!

More Exercise, Less Stress, Better Nutrition

One of those studies, conducted at the University of Medicine and Dentistry of New Jersey, involved 86 men (average age, 57) whose resting diastolic blood pressure (the second number of your blood pressure reading; like the 70 part of a 120/70) was 95 to 105 mmHg (millimeters of mercury). The men were assigned to two groups for three months of different treatments.

In one group, the men were given either 80 milligrams of the blood pressure–dropping drug propranolol twice daily or two placebo pills that looked like propranolol but contained no active drug. The men in the other group got no pills at all.

Instead, they exercised, modified their intake of salt, fat, and alcoholic beverages, and attended weekly stress management sessions. (The men in the drug-or-placebo group received no such counseling and made no changes in their diet or exercise habits.)

By the study's end, the men who had exercised, improved their diet, and reduced their stress had an average blood pressure reduction of nearly 13 mmHg, compared with only 8 mmHg for those on drug therapy!

Drugs Plus Exercise No Better Than Exercise Alone!

The other study, which caused quite a buzz in medical circles, was conducted at Johns Hopkins University. It looked at the effects of exercise alone and came up with a surprising finding.

Men who simply participated in an exercise program controlled their blood pressure just as well as men who worked out *and* took drugs to control their hypertension. The study involved 52 men aged 25 to 59, all with resting diastolic blood pressures between 90 and 105 mmHg.

The men were divided into three groups. Men in the

first group were given a beta-blocking drug to lower their blood pressure. Men in the second group took another type of antihypertension drug, a calcium channel blocker. The men in the third group got placebo pills that contained no active drug.

All of the men, however, took part in a ten-week exercise regimen that included weight training, walking, jogging, or cycling.

At the end of the study, the men taking the placebos had an average blood pressure of 131/84. Those taking the drugs didn't do any better. In fact, their averages of 138/88 and 132/88 were just a bit higher than the exercise-alone group.

These results certainly suggest that some mild hypertensives are able to control their blood pressure simply by enrolling in a good excercise program.

Johns Hopkins rehabilitation specialist Kerry Stewart, Ed.D., coinvestigator (with a cardiologist) on the study, adds that it may be possible for some men who are already taking drugs to gradually (under their doctor's supervision, of course) "wean" themselves off those drugs—or at least get by on lower doses.

Earlier Study Lends Support

Earlier research supports this positive outlook. A study published in the *Journal of the American Medical Association* reported that 40 percent of people studied (who had been taking drugs for years to keep their numbers down) were able to control their blood pressure with dietary changes and moderate exercise alone.

The author of that study, Rose Stamler, a professor of epidemiology at Chicago's Northwestern University Medical School, acknowledges the positive effects of exercise but stresses the benefits that good eating can convey on your blood pressure. "When blood pressure elevation is not too severe and there are no cardiovascular complications, an improved nutrition program may help maintain normal pressure without drugs—or at least allow people to reduce their dosage," she says.

PRESSURE POINTS: HOW TO LOWER YOUR BP THE DRUG-FREE WAY

Exactly *how* should you exercise? You could do worse than to follow the program put together for the Johns Hopkins study. They used walking, jogging, cycling, and swimming to control blood pressure.

You should, of course, discuss *any* new exercise program with your doctor first. Then, with his or her okay, you should perform whichever of those exercises appeals to you the most at least three times a week, for a continuous workout of 20 to 60 minutes each time.

(Remember, if you're already taking drugs to control your condition, don't stop until you work out the details with your doctor.)

Weight training can also be beneficial, but don't even *think* of doing it without your doctor's blessing, since blood pressure can undergo an extreme rise during such exercise.

As for diet, epidemiologist Rose Stamler of the Northwestern University Medical School believes that restricting salt intake is a major factor in blood pressure control. "People in the United States consume about ten times the amount of salt that they need," she says.

Cutting back on happy hour is also important. Stamler's close examination of at-risk populations has led her to believe that mild hypertensives should indulge in no more than two alcoholic drinks per day.

Caffeine has also been shown to raise blood pressure levels—especially in people who smoke.

Finally, if you're overweight, it's time to slim down! Stamler suggests you cut back on calories in general, and pay special attention to limiting your intake of saturated fats and cholesterol. That regular exercise program you're planning will help the pound-shedding process.

And don't be surprised if following these healthy tips generates a synergy of self-help that eases *all* of your life's pressures—not just the ones in your blood.

Such a drug-free approach, she points out, allows people with pressure problems "to avoid some of the unwanted side effects of those drugs, such as a rise in blood glucose or increased lipid levels." (Such rises could adversely affect people with diabetic tendencies or cholesterol problems.) Some blood pressure drugs have also been shown to cause sexual problems, including impotence.

But What about the *High* Guys?

Putting aside the pills in favor of working out and eating right is great news. But all the experts interviewed kept pointing out that they were talking *only* about "*mildly* hypertensive people," which basically refers to men with a diastolic reading of 90 to 105 or so.

So what about men with more severe high blood pressure? Won't they get *any* benefits from working out and eating better?

"We don't have the data to say with any certainty that people with more severe hypertension will be able to achieve *total* control of their condition with a diet and exercise program alone," explains epidemiologist Stamler.

But she feels that the data do indicate that such people may get considerable benefit—in terms of lowering their drug dosages and, in the long run, possibly even becoming drug free—if they adopt the right diet and exercise program.

Exercising and eating right will never make anyone's pressure worse, she says. And it's your best bet at controlling your blood pressure without the side effects that drugs can cause.

Super-Nutrient News

The Right Way to Get Your "A"

By Sheldon Saul Hendler, M.D., Ph.D.

When it comes to grabbing headlines, no nutrient can compete with vitamin A: "Low Vitamin A Intake Linked to Cancer," "Prevent Cancer: Eat Carrots," and "Vitamin A Curbs Lung Cancer in Smokers." The drumbeaters are not just megadose advocates. They include top researchers at the National Research Council and the National Cancer Institute. Everybody seems to be catching "carrot fever."

So, what's up, doc? There's no question that vitamin A—also known as retinol or beta-carotene, its biological precursor—is an essential nutrient. Among other things, we need it for reproduction, cell development, and vision (especially night vision). Vitamin A deficiency causes biological changes that resemble precancerous conditions, an observation that helped focus research attention on its role in cancer prevention.

Pros

Vitamin A (actually beta-carotene) is the pigment that gives many foods their yellow or orange color: carrots, sweet potatoes, cantaloupe, etc. Literally hundreds of scientific papers demonstrate that vitamin A has cancer-protective effects in animals, and studies of smokers show that those with the lowest beta-carotene intake are at greatest risk for lung cancer. Scientists believe beta-carotene helps prevent cancer by reducing cell damage caused by highly reactive oxygen ions known as free radicals or singlet oxygen. One group of researchers has called beta-carotene "the most efficient singlet oxygen [eliminator] thus far discovered."

Vitamin A also helps fight infection. In animal studies, vitamin A supplements have boosted immune system responsiveness. In humans, vitamin A deficiency is associated with a higher incidence of infection, and high doses of the vitamin markedly reduce the immune-suppressive effects of surgical anesthesia and cancer chemotherapy and radiation.

In addition, vitamin A spurs wound healing in laboratory animals. The incision wounds of diabetics recovering from surgery often heal very slowly. "We believe," researchers write, "that just as supplemental vitamin A improves immune function in traumatized animals, it will be especially useful in preventing wound infection and promoting wound healing in surgical diabetic patients."

Cons

On the other hand, high doses of fully formed vitamin A (i.e., not its precursor, beta-carotene) can cause headache, nausea, blurred vision, hair loss, itchy eyes, aching bones, and skin sores. How much is too much? That depends. Some people can take 50,000 international units (IU) a day for years with no problem, while others react to a single 20,000–international-unit capsule. Adverse reactions quickly clear up when the vitamin dose is reduced. However, no toxicity has been observed in people taking even very high doses of beta-carotene—500,000 international units a day.

In doses of 40,000 international units a day or more, fully formed vitamin A has also been linked to birth defects in the children of women who took it while pregnant. Beta-carotene has never been linked to birth defects—even at high doses. But pregnant women should not take any drug, vitamin, mineral, or food supplement without first consulting their physician.

Finally, fully formed vitamin A causes bone disease

among those with chronic kidney failure. People on dialysis should consult their physician before taking this vitamin.

Recommendations

The U.S. Recommended Daily Allowance (USRDA) for vitamin A is 5,000 international units. However, this dose may be insufficient. Some megavitamin advocates recommend up to 50,000 international units a day, but this dose of fully formed vitamin A would almost certainly cause toxicity in sensitive individuals.

Because beta-carotene provides the same benefits as vitamin A without the toxicity, there is no reason to take the fully formed vitamin (unless a physician prescribes it).

One average carrot contains about 5,000 international units of beta-carotene. A single sweet potato contains 10,000. Other foods rich in vitamin A include broccoli, spinach, cantaloupe, winter squash, papayas, apricots, watermelon, tomatoes, lettuce, fish-liver oils, and meats.

Beta-carotene supplements are widely available. I recommend 15,000 to 25,000 international units of beta-carotene supplementation a day.

Although adverse reactions to beta-carotene are highly unlikely, discontinue taking the supplement if any symptoms of toxicity develop.

High doses of beta-carotene can turn the palms yellow or orange (carotenoderma). This condition is benign and disappears when the vitamin is discontinued or reduced.

One final note: Vitamin E supplements in doses greater than 600 international units a day interfere with beta-carotene absorption and utilization.

The Calcium Connection

NEWS FLASH: Studies show that only a few Americans get 100 percent of the Recommended Dietary Allowance (RDA) for calcium. In fact, if you get even half the RDA, you're about average.

Although getting less than the RDA doesn't necessarily mean you're deficient (since RDAs are set a little higher than necessary for most people), experts are concerned. Especially since scientists are starting to uncover evidence that a lifetime of low calcium may contribute to our high rates of colon cancer and the bone-thinning disease called osteoporosis. A woman's chance of dying zooms by as much as 20 percent in the year after an osteoporosis-weakened hip fracture, and colon cancer claims over 60,000 lives a year. And for some hypertensives, low calcium levels may be complicating efforts to control their blood pressure. Uncontrolled hypertension makes you three times more likely to develop life-threatening heart disease. So the chance that calcium may cut the death toll from these diseases means this common mineral is getting a lot of attention in scientific circles these days. Here's what the latest research is telling us.

Heading Off a Bone Market Crash

Your skeleton is a calcium bank, and your body makes deposits into it and withdrawals from it. After menopause, when most osteoporosis occurs, withdrawals exceed deposits. Women who suffer broken vertebrae and hips are those whose accounts have gone into the red. (Osteoporosis affects men as well, although male hormones, larger bone size, and other factors give them some protection until their eighties or nineties.)

Getting enough calcium throughout life helps to hedge against this bone bankruptcy. For women, getting adequate calcium before menopause is especially important. The more calcium in their bank when they enter middle age (that is, the healthier their bones), the more they can afford to lose before they get into trouble. (Although getting more than 1,000 milligrams of calcium daily doesn't increase bone mass in premenopausal women.)

It's still not clear, though, whether dietary calcium can completely prevent osteoporosis. Studies looking at the question have come up with conflicting results. (Estrogen replacement after menopause, however, has been shown to prevent the disease in most women. And it's known that weight-bearing exercise—the kind you do upright, like walking and weight lifting—stimulates your bones toward greater strength.)

But there is growing evidence suggesting that if calcium can't bring bone loss to a standstill after menopause, it may at least slow it down.

The first solid study on this was completed in 1985 in Denmark. Thirty-six women past menopause were divided into three groups. During the two-year study, one group took estrogen, one took 2,000 milligrams of calcium a day, and one took blank pills (placebos). The results: The calcium group had less bone loss than the placebo group but more bone loss than those taking estrogen. And the calcium group experienced the least amount of bone loss in the long bone of the arms, compared to the spongy bone of the spine (*New England Journal of Medicine*).

Some later research also hinted that calcium may slow bone loss, and the Danish success was repeated here in the United States. Researchers at the University of Wisconsin, Madison, began with 169 women, ages 35 to 65. They gave half of them a supplement of 1,500 milligrams of calcium a day and the other half a blank pill. The researchers measured the women's rate of bone loss at a half-dozen places in their upper and lower arms 11 times over the next four years. This time taking extra calcium appeared to slow the rate at which postmenopausal women were losing bone mass at all six sites, while all the women on blank pills lost bone at a normal rate (*American Journal of Clinical Nutrition*).

The study's chief investigator, Everett Smith, Ph.D., believes that he can explain why calcium had such a poor showing in the other research. In some studies the time frame was too short, he says—subjects have to be watched for several years (or be increased in number) to see an effect from calcium. Other studies compared one group of women with another to see whether those with lower calcium intake had lower bone mass. That doesn't work, he says, because individuals vary so greatly in how they metabolize bone. You have to look at each woman over time to see whether adding calcium makes a difference in the way she loses bone.

Dr. Smith expects larger, long-term studies to confirm that dietary calcium is a good way to fight bone loss and osteoporosis. And in this research, scientists will be able to take advantage of new testing technology to monitor bone loss in women's spines and hips—primary fracture targets that were hard to measure in the past. Dual-energy x-ray photometry takes only 10 minutes and uses one-fifteenth the radiation of a chest x-ray.

Until the calcium/osteoporosis evidence is stronger, experts say that the smart thing to do is make sure you're getting the RDA for calcium. The RDA for males and females age 11 to 24 and for pregnant and lactating women is 1,200 milligrams daily. For older people, it's 800 milligrams. But for postmenopausal women at risk for osteoporosis who can't take estrogen, many calcium authorities recommend around 1,200 milligrams daily. (Risk factors include a family history of fractures, smoking, alcoholism, certain drug treatments, and early menopause.)

Calcium versus Colon Cancer

For several years, experts have suspected that calcium might be able to calm down the agitated growth of cells that's associated with cancer in our colon, the tail end of our intestines.

Researchers started by showing that, in rats, high-fat diets lead to an excess of bile acids and fatty acids in the colon. Rat colons respond to these irritants by growing new cells in the lining layer—a process called proliferation. It's also found in humans and thought to be a process that can increase during the development of colon cancer. And it was in rats that scientists discovered that extra calcium passing through the intestines seemed to stop the cell proliferation that bile acids and fatty acids caused.

Then in 1985 came the first study to explore the calcium-colon cancer link in humans. At the Memorial Sloan-Kettering Cancer Center in New York City, scientists chose as their subjects ten people who had colon cancer in their family—a strong predictor that they might get colon cancer themselves. The researchers gave their subjects 1,250 milligrams of calcium a day and took samples of their colon linings before and after treatment. After two to three months on calcium, cell proliferation had slowed by more than 40 percent (*New England Journal of Medicine*).

Later, scientists at the University of Utah School of Medicine in Salt Lake City produced some more evidence for the calcium/colon cancer theory. They compared 231 people diagnosed with colon cancer with 391 people without cancer. The scientists collected data on both groups' food intake for the two-year period before any cancer diagnosis, or before the end of the study. They found that people without colon cancer had a consistently higher intake of calcium than those diagnosed with the disease (*American Journal of Epidemiology*).

And now there's a study that seems to confirm the 1985 findings. It involves a larger group of people who either had a family history of colon cancer or had surgery to remove colon polyps, which tend to become cancerous over time. These people have slightly greater rates of cell proliferation in the colon than normal. Researchers at Ichilov Hospital in Israel gave 35 men and women 1,250 to 1,500 milligrams of calcium a day for three months and examined colon tissues removed from their subjects before, during, and after the treatment. Once again, abnormal cell proliferation dropped by 35.9 percent after one month, and returned to abnormally high rates after calcium treatment ended (*Gut*).

In both these cell-proliferation studies, by looking at the colon-lining samples under a microscope the researchers could see some amazing things. The shape of the colon lining's normal nooks and crannies (called "crypts") actually changed after calcium treatment. More normal cells had formed in a way that might protect the colon from attack by bile acids, and the number of abnormally formed cells had actually decreased. The resulting crypts then resembled those of Seventh-Day Adventist vegetarians, a group known for its low rates of colon and other types of cancer.

Martin Lipkin, M.D., one of the Memorial Sloan-Kettering Cancer Center researchers, offers some possible explanations for how calcium may stop abnormal cell proliferation. "If there is sufficient calcium in the colon, it may bind with bile acids and fatty acids in a way that keeps them out of contact with cells lining the colon, reducing proliferation," he says. "Or calcium itself may come into contact with the lining of cells and directly interfere with the abnormal proliferation."

Researchers point out that these studies are too small to draw firm conclusions yet and that stopping cell proliferation may or may not stop cancer. But the data have already inspired several larger, longer-term studies in which people at high risk of colon cancer are being given calcium.

Experimental Weapon against Hypertension

Studies of calcium's possible effect on high blood pressure have produced a roller coaster of results. Several studies suggested that calcium could reduce elevated blood pressure, while others found no effect. And, in at least one study, blood pressure went up when subjects consumed extra calcium.

Things started to make sense, though, after research suggested that only certain people might benefit from calcium and some might not—and that it may be possible to tell who was who. A 1986 study at New York Hospital-Cornell Medical Center showed that calcium works to lower blood pressure in the same people for whom dietary sodium tends to raise it (*Journal of Hypertension*). These people are called "salt sensitive." And about 60 percent of people with high blood pressure are estimated to fit this category. Then a 1988 study done at Purdue University found that, among other things, being older and having higher levels of parathyroid hormone made it more likely that calcium could have a pressure-lowering effect (*American Journal of Clinical Nutrition*).

Michael B. Zemel, Ph.D., associate professor of endocrinology and nutrition and food science at Wayne State University in Detroit, is one of the researchers helping to pin down who could benefit from adding extra calcium to their diet. He's done a series of studies in which calcium seemed to lower blood pressure in African-Americans and the elderly—two groups known to be salt sensitive (*American Journal of Hypertension*).

There are actually two possible explanations of how calcium might be able to reduce blood pressure levels, says Dr. Zemel. The simple one goes like this: In salt-sensitive people, eating too much salt makes them retain water. That causes the amount of water in their blood vessels to go up, raising pressure just like turning up the flow through a garden hose. That's why diuretics—drugs to make your body release water—lower blood pressure for some people. Calcium seems to help your kidneys release sodium and water, so you get a natural diuretic effect. (Dr. Zemel cautions that calcium is not a substitute for prescribed diuretics, and you should not stop taking any blood pressure medication on your own without first talking it over with your doctor.)

The second theory ties in the role of the parathyroid hormone that was identified in the earlier Purdue study, says Dr. Zemel. Just as calcium helps salt-sensitive people lose excess sodium, too much salt causes them to lose calcium from their blood. When this happens, the body responds by releasing parathyroid hormone plus another hormone derived from the vitamin D we get from food. Together, these two hormones push more calcium into the smooth muscle cells lining the blood vessels (taking it out of bone storage). When it's inside these cells, calcium's job is to force the muscles to contract, which raises the blood pressure just like a hand squeezing tightly around a garden hose. But calcium we eat acts to prevent the release of the parathyroid and vitamin D hormones so no calcium is pushed into smooth muscle cells. Your blood vessels stay relaxed and blood pressure stays down (*Journal of Laboratory and Clinical Medicine*).

Dr. Zemel expects that future studies of calcium targeting salt-sensitive people will show more consistent results than the earlier research that used a hit-or-miss ap-

Calcium Foods: How Much Do You Need?

One glass of milk a day won't do it. To meet your RDA for calcium, you'll need to drink—or eat—a whole lot more of calcium-packed foods. For example, to get 1,000 milligrams of calcium you'd need $3\frac{1}{3}$ 8-ounce glasses of milk, or 22 sardines (with bones), or 48 $\frac{1}{2}$-cup servings of broccoli.

But don't get discouraged. You can get all the calcium you need by choosing wisely from a wide variety of foods, some of which are listed in the accompanying table. By including several of these in daily menus, you can easily meet your calcium RDA.

Food/Portion	Calcium (mg)
Dairy Products	
Cheese	
Cottage, low-fat (1%), $\frac{1}{2}$ cup	69
Mozzarella, skim milk, 1 oz.	183
Ricotta, skim milk, $\frac{1}{2}$ cup	335
Swiss, 1 oz.	272
Milk, nonfat, fluid, 1 cup	302
Yogurt, 1 cup*	
Low-fat, plain	415
Nonfat, plain	452
Legumes	
Lentils, whole, cooked, 1 cup*	50
Soybeans, cooked, 1 cup	131
Tempeh, 1 cup	154
Tofu, 1 piece, 4.2 oz.	154
Nuts and Seeds	
Brazil nuts, 1 oz.	50
Pistachio nuts, 1 oz.*	38
Sesame seeds, 1 oz.	281
Seafood	
Bass, black, baked, 3 oz.	72
Mackerel, canned, 3 oz.	205
Sardines, canned in oil, 3 oz. (7 fish)*	322
Vegetables	
Broccoli, boiled, 1 cup*	178
Collard greens, frozen, boiled, 1 cup	357
Kale, frozen, boiled, 1 cup	179

*By eating just these five foods in a single day you'll get more than 1,000 milligrams of calcium.

proach of testing anyone with high blood pressure. He says research is needed to establish optimum calcium intake and whether calcium may help people who must use blood pressure medications to minimize the amount of drugs they need. Even now a major study at ten research centers includes calcium among the nutritional and lifestyle changes being tested for effects on lowering blood pressure.

The Prudent Calcium Course

Many researchers agree: In light of all the evidence, the best course for everyone is to try to get the RDA for calcium by eating lots of calcium-rich foods (see "Calcium Foods: How Much Do You Need?" on page 105).

Six Tips for the Lactose Intolerant

Sure, it's harder to get your Recommended Dietary Allowance for calcium if dairy foods leave you feeling gassy and bloated. But there are ways around lactose intolerance—an inability to properly digest the milk sugar lactose. Try some of these proven alternatives from the National Dairy Council.

1. Combine your dairy food with dinner. Lactose is easier to digest when mixed with other foods.

2. Eat smaller servings throughout the day. For instance, take small drinks of milk with each meal instead of downing an entire glass at once. Your body may be able to manage the lactose in installments.

3. Add cocoa to your low-fat milk. Although they still don't know why, researchers have shown that cocoa makes milk more digestible.

4. Stick to yogurt. Helpful bacteria in yogurt digest the lactose for you.

5. Select only cheeses aged six months or longer, like Swiss or Cheddar. Aging removes most of the lactose from cheese.

6. Try liquid or tablet forms of lactase (available in drug stores), the milk-sugar–digesting enzyme that you're lacking, or milk that's made with lactase already added.

Many experts also say that if you're unable to eat enough calcium-containing foods, maybe because you can't digest dairy products, you may want to consider a supplement (see "Six Tips for the Lactose Intolerant" on page 106). Just keep in mind, calcium intake that goes too much over the RDA might be a problem for those who are susceptible to forming kidney stones.

B_{12}: More Than a Shot in the Dark

No energy? Appetite under par? Can't remember the very thing you promised yourself you wouldn't forget?

Vague complaints like these can suggest a wide variety of health problems, including a B_{12} deficiency. But it's a rare blood test that detects such a deficiency. So, say doctors, B_{12} injections are hardly ever warranted.

Now two studies challenge that point of view. They suggest that for some people with "normal" blood tests, B_{12} supplementation may be more than a shot in the dark. It may offer relief from a wide variety of complaints, including fatigue, memory loss, and even incontinence.

A Vital Vitamin

What exactly is B_{12}? Otherwise known as cyanocobalamin, it's important for normal growth, blood formation, and a healthy nervous system. Vitamin B_{12} plays an integral part in the formation of blood cells. Without it, red blood cell production decreases. The result of this B_{12} bombshell: anemia (which starves the body of oxygen, causing tiredness), bleeding, or infections.

Also, the vitamin quite literally keeps you from losing your nerve. B_{12} helps produce myelin, the protective coating that surrounds the nerves, much like rubber encases electrical wiring. Without myelin, nerves slowly deteriorate, causing a potpourri of neuropsychiatric problems. Feet can turn numb and tingle. You can have trouble walking or difficulty feeling the floor. The nerve damage can bring on the more subtle mental changes of the B_{12} blues—depression, confusion, and loss of memory.

Surprisingly, B_{12} deficiency usually isn't the result of ingesting too little B_{12} (the Recommended Dietary Allowance is only 3 micrograms, which most people easily get with their normal diet). More often, it's caused by an absorption problem.

With aging, the stomach can lose its ability to produce intrinsic factor, a substance that allows B_{12} to be absorbed in the small intestine. That's why B_{12}-deficient people usually need to take shots—to circumvent the digestive system.

In Search of B_{12}

The question is, how could some people who are presumed not to have B_{12} deficiency actually benefit from a B_{12} boost?

To understand, we must first look at how doctors determine B_{12} deficiency. Many physicians expect B_{12} deficiency to cause blood abnormalities long before it causes nerve damage (except in rare instances). So they often discount B_{12} deficiency if tests show normal blood, says Robert H. Allen, M.D., director of hematology, University of Colorado Health Sciences Center.

In one study, however, Dr. Allen and colleagues looked at 323 patients who suffered from B_{12} deficiency and discovered that 141 had symptoms of nerve damage. Contrary to traditional medical thinking, 40 of the 141 patients (28 percent) were found not to have the expected blood abnormalities (*New England Journal of Medicine*).

"I think the most important thing this study shows is that many of the standard teachings about B_{12} deficiency are wrong," says Dr. Allen.

In another study, from the University of Southern California (USC), 23 of 70 patients with B_{12} deficiency (33 percent) didn't have noticeable blood problems. Ralph Carmel, M.D., author of the study, concludes, "The experience at our hospital suggests that true [B₁₂] deficiency is more common than is currently appreciated" (*Archives of Internal Medicine*).

Another part of the problem, doctors say, is the way B₁₂ is measured. The standard test for B₁₂ was modified in 1978. The reason was that the test was discovered to react to some compounds that are similar to but are not B₁₂, creating false high B₁₂ readings. "A lot of cases of B₁₂ deficiency were missed because of that," says William S. Beck, M.D., professor of medicine at Harvard Medical School and director of hematology research at Massachusetts General Hospital. "Testing methods were corrected, so that's no longer a problem."

Now the problem seems to be what doctors expect to find when they measure B₁₂ serum levels (in the blood)—the first test for determining deficiency. The normal range for B₁₂ in the blood is about 200 to 900 picograms per milliliter (pg/ml). Most medical textbooks teach that true deficiency is based on finding serum B₁₂ levels of less than 100. But in Dr. Allen's study, 18 of the 40 deficient patients without blood abnormalities had levels between 100 and 200 (slightly low), and two actually had normal B₁₂ readings. This is why their B₁₂ deficiency could easily have been overlooked. Slightly low or low normal levels could have been dismissed as lab errors, as not worth investigating in this age of medical cost consciousness (especially when the expected anemia or other blood abnormalities weren't present). In the USC study, only 45 of the 70 deficient patients had the very low serum levels expected with B₁₂ deficiency.

Also, although Dr. Allen and others use 200 picograms per milliliter as a benchmark for B₁₂ deficiency, the exact number can vary from lab to lab.

The bright note to all this is that B₁₂ deficiency now seems to become apparent on lab tests at an earlier stage than many doctors have thought. Leading researchers now believe that many cases of B₁₂ deficiency can be detected before they even begin to cause serious damage. And that's important because the quicker the problem is caught, the more likely it is to be reversed.

Surprising Symptoms

And the B_{12} deficiency symptoms may be more numerous than many experts realize. In Dr. Allen's study, the patients had reported a total of 212 problems related to nerve damage, including abnormal gait, impaired touch or pain perception, decreased reflexes, and memory loss. After receiving B_{12} injections, 119 of the problems were completely resolved and 59 were partially resolved. In all, no improvement was shown for only eight of the problems attributed to lack of B_{12}. And all of the participants who completed the study showed at least some progress.

The list of problems that disappeared after B_{12} injections was not only long but also included some surprises—hallucinations, eye disorders, and incontinence. "Most people would never associate incontinence with B_{12} deficiency," says Dr. Allen.

"How common is this? I can't put a number on it, and I wouldn't say it was very common. But I recently read an article in the *New England Journal of Medicine* about incontinence, and it didn't even mention B_{12} deficiency as a possible cause," he says.

Victor Herbert, M.D., professor of medicine at Mt. Sinai and Veterans Administration Bronx Medical Centers and a leading B_{12} researcher, says he and others wrote about the association between B_{12} deficiency and problems such as incontinence way back in the 1950s.

Why these symptoms are seldom linked to B_{12} deficiency nowadays is illustrated by Dr. Allen's study. Although there was a control group, it's difficult to know how many of these patients would have improved without B_{12} injections—and, therefore, how many symptoms weren't caused by deficiency. Many of these psychological problems are vague, waxing and waning, so they're hard to measure scientifically. These technical problems have long vexed B_{12} researchers and may be why symptoms that Dr.

Herbert wrote about more than 30 years ago are still not included in some medical review articles.

Testing for B_{12}

So in light of all this, when should you have a B_{12} serum test? Consider being tested

• As soon as you exhibit unexplained nerve or blood problems of the kind that are seen in B_{12} deficiency. If your serum B_{12} level is below 300, Dr. Allen recommends an additional test—available commercially through several national labs. This test measures blood elements called metabolites. These elements (specifically methylmalonic acid and total homocysteine) increase in blood when B_{12} is deficient. If your symptoms strongly suggest B_{12} deficiency, Dr. Allen believes this additional test should be done even when the serum B_{12} level is above 300.
• At age 60, whether or not you show signs of deficiency, Dr. Herbert says. If your serum level is low or low normal, you should have another screening within three to six months. Based on that, you can determine with your doctor whether or not you need B_{12} supplementation.

The Placebo Effect

Although he believes that more research like Dr. Allen's is needed, Dr. Beck raised an intriguing question in his editorial accompanying the study: "Could it be that the many [B_{12}] injections given over the years for vague symptoms were in fact justified?" Perhaps. But although there is much confusion in the B_{12} field, experts agree on this point: There is no biological reason B_{12} should give you a boost or any other benefit if you don't have a deficiency. It's also not a one-time cure; if you need extra B_{12} now, you're going to need it for the rest of your life. So there's no point in getting B_{12} injections without being tested for deficiency. "Otherwise, at best, you're wasting your money," says Dr. Herbert.

Getting Your B₁₂

For all the hoopla over B_{12}, you need surprisingly little of it—one-ten-millionth of an ounce daily. In fact, it's pretty hard not to get enough B_{12} in your diet. (Remember, B_{12} deficiency is usually due to stomach problems that prevent the vitamin from being absorbed.)

The Trouble with Tempeh

Vegetarians had long thought they could get sufficient vitamin B_{12} in tempeh, a type of fermented soybean. The tempeh culture itself didn't produce B_{12}, but it was believed to carry bacterial microorganisms that did. But experts have concluded that's not so.

"Until recently, most tempeh manufacturers would not only make B_{12} claims on the nutritional panel, they would also have some sort of label that said 'Rich in B_{12}' or 'Vegetarian Source of B_{12},' " says Michael Cohen, president of Lightlife Food, a Greenfield, Massachusetts, company that's one of the nation's largest producers of tempeh. "It was a major marketing point for tempeh manufacturers and one we had to let go of because we really couldn't stand behind it."

The new view of tempeh is due in part to better testing. Tests that originally determined that B_{12} was in tempeh have been found to be detecting other substances. It may also be the case that the industry's improved hygienic techniques have destroyed the B_{12}-carrying bacteria that were once in these foods. "If vegetables do contain B_{12}, that's an indirect way of saying they're contaminated with helpful bacteria," says Robert H. Allen, M.D., of the University of Colorado Health Sciences Center. "When vegetarians from India moved to England . . . B_{12} problems increased because the food was less contaminated with bacteria."

So, experts say, strict vegetarians should take a B_{12} supplement, which can be in pill form, since presumably they would have no trouble absorbing the vitamin.

B_{12} is found only in animal products, such as meats (particularly liver), eggs, and milk. "If it swims, flies, or runs, it has B_{12}," says Dr. Herbert. Only strict vegetarians (and especially their newborn offspring) need be concerned about B_{12} deficiency through diet. But even for vegetarians, it takes a long time—perhaps ten years or more—to become deficient, because the body stores B_{12} in abundance.

New Light on Vitamin D

Until less than a century ago, life was timed by the daily and seasonal comings and goings of the sun. But now we hold the night at bay with street signs and track lighting, making our own timetables.

Or do we? Walter E. Stumpf, Ph.D., of the University of North Carolina, thinks it is likely that many of our physiologic rhythms are still influenced by light and dark.

Dr. Stumpf bases his theory, published in the journal *Psychopharmacology,* on findings made in the course of his landmark work of mapping the human nervous system. He discovered that there are receptors for vitamin D, the "sunshine" vitamin, in virtually all the systems of the body. Dr. Stumpf believes they must be there for a reason, and he speculates that the sun has acted, through millions of years of evolution, as a timekeeper, triggering some biological processes (eating, sleeping, and sex, for example) at their optimal times. (Vitamin D is called the sunshine vitamin, because our skin, liver, and kidneys use chemical processes triggered by sun exposure to make it.)

Vitamin D, in other words, may be one of the keys to how our internal body clock works. Current medical thinking assigns vitamin D a more modest role—ensuring that calcium is in balance in our blood, tissues, and organs, as well as keeping our bones solid. But Dr. Stumpf speculates that it drives the whole endocrine—hormonal—system, which regulates things as varied as insulin levels, hormonal secretions, and blood pressure. Vitamin D may even bear on our mental health, which could help explain seasonal affective disorder (SAD), or winter depression.

What makes Dr. Stumpf's theory still more intriguing is that science has discovered that vitamin D is itself a hormone, and as such is used in an entirely different, more cyclic pattern than other vitamins.

A New Name

As part of his theory, Dr. Stumpf has dubbed the form of vitamin D we need—1,25-dihydroxyvitamin D_3—"soltriol," in recognition of its origins with the sun and its hormonal function. And he thinks that all those vitamin D receptors he found in various parts of the body, including the intestines and reproductive system, reflect millions of years of evolution when people lived their entire lives by the timing of the sun.

Soltriol, he believes, keeps us in sync with the sun, perhaps triggering the release of thyroid-stimulating hormone, insulin, and digestive acids in the stomach at the optimal times.

But vitamin D does not work alone, he speculates. Rather, it's part of an "endocrinology of light and dark" that is balanced by melatonin, a substance secreted by the pineal gland, that is sometimes called the "hormone of darkness." Not much is known about the pineal gland, a tiny organ in the brain. In fact, melatonin was only discovered in the early 1970s. Melatonin's function in the body is still largely unknown, but one thing is for sure: Its levels in the blood follow a 24-hour rhythm and are highest during the night. Dr. Stumpf feels that if there are processes tied to sun, then there are surely counterprocesses that are controlled by the time we spend in darkness.

Dr. Stumpf's ideas are so new that they have not yet been examined by other researchers, and he himself admits that it may take a long time to verify his theories. Another stumbling block is that vitamin D is not widely studied in this country. So the question of whether or not the sun is the power behind our biological clock is probably not going to be answered until sometime in the 21st century.

Eat Right for Life

How to Love the Food That's Good for You

By George L. Blackburn, M.D., Ph.D.

New Year's resolutions are full of healthful intentions: to walk 3 miles a day; to floss daily (without fail); to lose 10 pounds in so many weeks; and, most challenging of all, to adopt the kind of low-fat, high-fiber diet that can take pounds off and add years to your life (even if it does mean giving up the foods you love and think you can't live without).

Actually, the last resolution isn't as tough as it sounds. The fact is, we don't eat the foods we love; we love the foods we eat.

If you had an Eastern European upbringing, for example, your palate may be accustomed to schnitzel and strudel. Does that mean you can't possibly be happy eating anything less? No, it simply means that through years of repetitive feedings, your taste buds have become programmed to expect those familiar flavors and textures. The good news is you can retrain your palate to accept leaner, healthier fare—and in a surprisingly short period of time.

Perhaps you've already taken a few steps to improve your diet. Maybe you've graduated from whole milk to low-fat to skim. Or you might have cut back your sodium intake. Or you've started eating more high-fiber foods. If you've maintained your new habit for a couple months, you've probably lost your taste for the previous foods. Whole milk now tastes like heavy cream to you; salted soups are far too salty for your taste; and you wouldn't think of skipping your afternoon fruit snack.

Actually, you can notice a difference in your food preference after just a week of retraining. Spa-goers know this firsthand. Checking into a health spa requires that you give up a lot of favorites. Gone are the croissants, the cheeseburger and fries, the Dove Bars. In their place: whole grain breads, lean meats and fish, brown rice—perhaps some frozen (nonfat) yogurt, if you're lucky. Water and fruit juices are the drinks of choice, edging out soda pop, beer, and wine. For snacking, air-popped popcorn, fruit, frozen low-fat yogurt pops, and sorbets replace salty potato chips.

If the new diet is unfamiliar to you, it will drive you bananas at first. But amazingly, after a few days you'll begin to appreciate the subtle flavors and bold textures of healthy food. By week's end, your palate will start to readjust. Cravings for fat, sodium, and sweets will gradually diminish. You'll actually prefer wholesome foods—at least for a short period after you return home.

A Palate-Retraining Program

If you don't believe me, try it yourself. Commit yourself to eating a truly healthy diet for just one week. This means a good breakfast, a wholesome main meal, a second light meal, and one or two snacks a day. I suggest you make a contract with yourself to follow through. Put it in writing. Tell your friends and family members how you plan to change your diet. It's harder to break diet restrictions that others are expecting you to keep. After you've signed your contract, carefully choose your meals for the week. It's important to do this in advance so you've got a definite plan to follow. Last-minute mealtime decisions can test your willpower.

Choose some exemplary breakfasts, lunches, and dinners. By this I mean meals that are low in fat (no more than 9 grams per entrée), with lots of high-fiber and nutrient-rich fruits, vegetables, and whole grains.

Keep your choices simple. In fact, you need only five menus to get you through the week: one well-balanced breakfast such as a whole grain cereal with fruit and skim milk, two lunches, and three dinners. I suggest your dinner entrées include one broiled or baked chicken dish, one pasta dish, and one vegetable dish (that is, a large plate of steamed vegetables). Don't worry about getting bored with your limited selections. Just choose from among your healthy favorites, make sure the recipes are easy to prepare, and make use of no-salt flavor enhancers like spices and dry mustard. These dishes will be the foundation of your on-the-healthy-side program.

A few other tips: Avoid eating out unless you're sure the restaurant serves low-fat meals. Say good-bye to soft drinks; drink skim milk, juices, and water instead. Snack on fresh fruit and the new healthy microwavable soups. Say no to creamery butter and yes to fruit butters. Have large salads. Do make sure you eat enough! The idea here is not to starve yourself (although you will probably lose weight as a natural consequence of low-fat eating)—it's to eat nutrient-laden healthy foods.

By the end of the week, see if you don't feel more energized and sleep better. Chances are, your cravings for unhealthy foods will be reduced, too.

Renew Your Contract

Unfortunately, one week isn't long enough to ingrain you to healthy eating habits for life. It's just enough to give you a taste of what, with a little more effort, could become a lifelong habit.

So now's the time to renew your contract with yourself—this time for a two- to four-week period. Add some additional low-fat, high-nutrition dishes to your repertoire. Keep in mind that the longer you stick with this palate-retraining program, the longer the results are likely to last. Of course, at some point, your taste buds will probably start to drift again. So I suggest a refresher course for two weeks every six months or so. Or take your vacation at a health spa. You'll be back on track in no time.

Your Personal Diet Makeover

By Judith S. Stern, Sc.D., R.D., and
   Liz Applegate, Ph.D.

How's your diet? Sure, you try to eat right most of the time. But if you're like most people, you've probably wondered whether you're really succeeding in eating the way you should for optimal health.

Now you can find out for sure. In just three days, you can have a clearer understanding of your nutrition habits—what you're doing right, and where there's room for improvement—with this do-it-yourself diet analysis.

This inquiry will take you through a process similar to the one you'd go through if you would consult with a professional dietitian/nutritionist.

First, you'll write down everything you eat for three days. Then, using that information, you'll take an eye-opening quiz that'll help you pinpoint your nutritional strengths and weaknesses. The questions focus on important areas: key vitamins and minerals; fat; fiber; sodium; and the "empty foods," like sweets. After the quiz, there's some solid advice on getting—or keeping—your diet on track. The recommendations are based, in part, on the National Research Council's latest report on diet and health.

This self-test, of course, can't track your diet nearly as precisely as a professionally supervised analysis. So don't hesitate to consult a professional dietitian/nutritionist, especially if you have health problems, are pregnant, are on a low-calorie or restricted diet, or if the quiz uncovers some dietary trouble spots that you want to investigate further.

But if you're a healthy, active adult ready to fine-tune your diet for maximum nutrition and health, get yourself a pencil and a notebook and start this week!

Step #1: Filling Out Your Food Diary

Pick three consecutive days in a week in which your eating habits are fairly typical. (Don't choose a week when you're on vacation!) Ideally, you should include one weekend day. For instance, you can record on a Sunday, Monday, and Tuesday, or a Thursday, Friday, and Saturday.

• Don't change your eating habits for this diary, or try to be "good" during the three days: An accurate record will be the most helpful to you.
• Write down everything you eat during the three days, including seasonings, beverages, and snacks. Note how the foods are prepared. Look over the quiz before you start, to see what kinds of questions you'll be asked. That'll help you know what other information you need to record.
• Try to be precise about serving sizes, using measuring cups and a food scale if necessary.
• Carry a small notebook and pencil with you each day for your diary keeping. It's better to write things down right after meals than to try to remember later.

Step #2: Taking the Quiz

As you read each question, review your food diary and circle the appropriate answer. Circle only one answer for each question. You may be asked to average the number of servings per day (add up the number over three days and divide by three), or to give the total number of servings you ate in the three days. If you're uncertain, use an estimate.

• Pay attention to serving sizes described in the question. For example, if a serving of vegetables is described as $\frac{1}{2}$ cup and you ate 1 cup, count it as two servings.
• At the end of each section, add up the points assigned to each answer and write down the total. (Negative points should be subtracted from the section's score.)
• Add up all the section scores to get an overall score.

Section I: Vitamins and Minerals

1. About how many servings of grain products did you eat each day? (Use an average figure. One serving = one slice

of bread; or ½ cup cooked grain, such as pasta, rice, or barley; or ½ cup of dry cereal.) Do not include high-fat/high-sugar biscuits, croissants, cookies, cakes, and so forth.

a. 6 or more/1 day (5 points)
b. 4 to 5 (4 points)
c. 3 (2 points)
d. 1 to 2 (1 point)
e. none (0 points)

2. About how many servings of high-calcium foods (like milk, yogurt, cheese, tofu, and canned salmon) did you eat each day? (Use an average. One serving = 1 cup milk or yogurt, 1 ounce cheese, ½ cup canned salmon, or 4 ounces tofu.)

a. 3 or more/1 day (5 points)
b. 2 (4 points)
c. 1 (3 points)
d. none (−1 point)

3. About how many servings of dark green leafy vegetables did you eat each day? These include kale, collard greens, dark green leaf lettuce, and others. (Use an average. One serving = 1 cup raw or ½ cup cooked.)

a. 2 or more/1 day (5 points)
b. 1 (4 points)
c. ½ (3 points)
d. none (0 points)

4. Over three days, how many servings of orange or yellow vegetables or fruit did you eat? These include winter squash, pumpkins, carrots, melons, peaches, and apricots. (One serving = ½ cup cooked, or 1 cup raw, or ½ cup juice.)

a. 3 or more/3 days (5 points)
b. 2 (3 points)
c. 1 (2 points)
d. none (0 points)

5. How many servings of citrus fruits or other fruits high in vitamin C (like strawberries) did you eat during three days? (One serving = 1 piece, or ½ cup juice, or 1 cup raw.)

a. 3 or more/3 days (4 points)
b. 2 (3 points)
c. 1 (2 points)
d. none (0 points)

6. How many servings of cruciferous vegetables did you eat during three days? Cruciferous vegetables include broccoli, cauliflower, cabbage, brussels sprouts, bok choy, turnips, and rutabaga. (One serving = $\frac{1}{2}$ cup cooked or 1 cup raw.)

a. 3 or more/3 days (4 points)

b. 2 (3 points)

c. 1 (2 points)

d. none (0 points)

7. Did you eat at least one 3-ounce serving of lean red meat, or two 3-ounce servings of chicken or turkey, during the three-day period?

a. yes (2 points)

b. no (0 points)

Section I Score:

Section II: Fats

8. What did you usually spread on your bread, toast, rolls, or muffins?

a. butter, cream cheese (-2 points)

b. margarine (0 points)

c. jam (2 points)

d. fruit spread or nothing (3 points)

9. What type of dairy products (milk, cottage cheese, yogurt, and so forth) did you usually eat or drink?

a. cream, half-and-half, full-fat ice cream (-3 points)

b. whole milk (-1 point)

c. 2 percent fat (2 points)

d. 1 percent fat (3 points)

e. nonfat or skim (4 points)

10. During the three-day span, how many times did you eat processed meats, such as bacon, luncheon meats, sausage, frankfurters, or salami?

a. 3 or more/3 days (-5 points)

b. 2 (-2 points)

c. 1 (1 point)

d. none (3 points)

11. Did you always remove skin from poultry and trim visible fat from meats?

a. yes (4 points)

b. no (−3 points)

12. Over three days, how many times did you eat processed crackers, chips or commercially baked goods, or homemade high-fat cakes and cookies?

a. 5 or more/3 days (−2 points)

b. 3 to 4 (0 points)

c. 1 to 2 (2 points)

d. none (4 points)

13. When preparing meals or eating out, how many times during three days were foods fried in oil, sautéed in butter or margarine, prepared or served with mayonnaise, tartar sauce, or other fatty dressings or sauces?

a. 5 or more/3 days (−3 points)

b. 3 to 4 (−1 point)

c. 1 to 2 (2 points)

d. none (4 points)

14. What type of dressing do you usually put on your salad?

a. regular salad dressing or oil and vinegar (−1 point)

b. reduced calorie, i.e., low-fat dressing (3 points)

c. lemon juice, tomato juice, or vinegar (4 points)

d. none (4 points)

15. Did you eat more than two 3-ounce servings of meat on any day?

a. yes (−1 point)

b. no (2 points)

16. Did you eat more than 2 ounces of full-fat cheese on any day? Full-fat cheeses may include Cheddar, Swiss, Brie, Jack, and others.

a. yes (−1 point)

b. no (2 points)

Section II Score:

Section III: Types of Fat

17. When you used fat or oil for cooking, did you usually use:

a. butter or hard margarine (−1 point)

b. a combination of butter/vegetable oil (0 points)

c. margarine, soft tub; regular or reduced calorie (2 points)

d. oils high in polyunsaturated fatty acids: soy, safflower, corn (3 points)

e. oils high in monounsaturated fats: olive, canola (4 points)

18. About how many egg yolks did you eat during the three-day period? (Include yolks in baked products and casseroles, as well as egg dishes like scrambled eggs.)

a. 3 or more/3 days (− 1 point)

b. 2 (0 points)

c. 1 (1 point)

d. none (2 points)

19. During the three days, did you eat processed foods made with fats that are high in saturated fatty acids? (The label will say palm or coconut oil, or butter; these are typically found in commercially made cookies, granola bars, and crackers.)

a. yes (0 points)

b. no (3 points)

Section III Score:

Section IV: Fiber

20. What type of bread (including rolls and muffins) did you usually eat?

a. whole wheat, whole grain (4 points)

b. white or partial whole wheat (2 points)

21. How many servings of oat products did you average daily? (One serving = 1 cup cooked oatmeal or oat bran.)

a. 2 or more/1 day (4 points)

b. 1 (3 points)

c. ½ (2 points)

d. none (0 points)

22. How many times during the three-day period did you eat beans (legumes), such as kidney beans, pintos, garbanzos, soybeans, lentils, and split peas?

a. 3 or more/3 days (4 points)

b. 2 (3 points)

c. 1 (2 points)

d. none (0 points)

23. How many times during the three-day period did you eat high-fiber breakfast cereals?
a. 3 or more/3 days (4 points)
b. 2 (3 points)
c. 1 (2 points)
d. none (0 points)

24. How many times during the three-day period did you eat cooked whole grain side dishes, such as brown rice or barley?
a. 3 or more/3 days (4 points)
b. 2 (3 points)
c. 1 (2 points)
d. none (0 points)

25. Approximately how many servings of canned or fresh fruits and vegetables did you eat every day? (Use an average. One serving = $\frac{1}{2}$ cup cooked or 1 cup or one piece raw.)
a. 7 or more/1 day (5 points)
b. 5 to 6 (4 points)
c. 3 to 4 (2 points)
d. 1 to 2 (1 point)
e. none (-2 points)

Section IV Score:

Section V: Sodium

26. About how many servings of high-sodium processed foods did you consume each day, on average? (One serving = 1 cup canned food such as soup, 3 ounces luncheon meats, or $\frac{1}{2}$ cup commercially baked goods such as crackers.)
a. 4 or more/1 day (-1 point)
b. 2 to 3 (1 point)
c. 0 to 1 (5 points)

27. What seasonings do you typically add to foods?
a. garlic, herbs, lemon juice, no-salt spices (5 points)
b. salt substitute (3 points)
c. soy sauce, garlic or onion salt, teriyaki sauce (-1 point)
d. salt (-1 point)

Section V Score:

Section VI: "Empty" Foods

28. How many servings of alcoholic drinks did you consume, on the average, daily? (One serving = 12 ounces beer, 4 ounces wine, or 1 ounce liquor.)
a. 2 or more/1 day (− 5 points)
b. 1/1 day (− 3 points)
c. 1 to 2/week (− 1 point)
d. none (5 points)

29. What beverage did you most frequently drink with meals or snacks?
a. water, mineral water, or seltzer (5 points)
b. nonfat skim milk (5 points)
c. fruit juice (3 points)
d. diet soda (1 point)
e. fruit drink or soda (0 points)
f. coffee/tea (0 points)

30. How many servings of caffeine-containing beverages did you drink daily? (One serving = 6 ounces coffee, 10 ounces tea, 12 ounces soda.)
a. 3 or more (− 2 points)
b. 2 (0 points)
c. 1 (1 point)
d. none (2 points)

31. How many times did you eat high-sugar, high-calorie foods during the three-day period (pie, cake, candy, chocolate, cookies, ice cream)?
a. 5 to 6 or more/3 days (− 3 points)
b. 3 to 4 (0 points)
c. 1 to 2 (2 points)
d. none (5 points)

Section VI Score:

Section VII: Behavior

32. Are you 10 or more pounds over the weight you'd like to be?
a. yes (0 points)
b. no (5 points)

33. Do you eat regularly during the day, rarely or never skipping meals?
a. yes (1 point)
b. no (0 points)
34. How many times do you snack daily?
a. 3 or more (−2 points)
b. 2 (0 points)
c. 1 (1 point)
d. none (3 points)

Section VII Score:

Total Quiz Score:

How Did You Do?

The separate scores for each section can give you the best idea of how you're eating. Here's what your scores mean.

Section I • If you scored more than 22 points, you're probably eating an abundance of vitamin- and mineral-rich foods. If you scored under 22 points, see below for ways to improve. Regardless of your total score for this section, be sure to pay particular attention to your points on questions 2 and 7.

Section II • If your score is over 20, your fat intake is probably reasonable. If it's under 20, consider reducing fat further. Authorities agree that cutting fat is America's number one nutritional priority for reducing risk of heart disease and possibly some forms of cancer and obesity.

Section III • If your score is under 5, you may need to choose your fats more wisely. The type as well as the quantity of fat can affect health.

Section IV • If your score is over 20, your fiber intake is probably excellent. The regular use of fiber-rich, whole grain products improves bowel function, may reduce blood cholesterol, and possibly protects against certain forms of cancer. It's important to get both soluble and insoluble fiber. Soluble fiber (found in oats, beans, and apples) may help lower blood-cholesterol levels. Insoluble fiber (found in whole wheat and vegetables) assists bowel function.

Section V • If your score is under 8, consider steps to reduce sodium. About a third of people who have high blood pressure can decrease their pressure significantly by restricting sodium intake.

Section VI • Over 10 points is excellent, 5 points is fair, under 3 is cause for concern. The "empty foods" in your diet provide mostly calories and few nutrients, or may actually harm your nutritional status.

Section VII • Obesity can increase risk of chronic disease. So if your score is over 5, meaning you're not overweight, congratulations—you either chose the right parents or you're doing something right. If you are overweight, you may find that changing certain behaviors can help, along with paying special attention to your intake of fats and sugar.

Your total quiz score (maximum possible points: 136) tells you how your diet rates overall.

Over 100 • Outstanding! You scored high in every section, which means your diet is probably excellent.

80 to 100 • Pretty good. Look at your problem areas and make the changes you need.

60 to 79 • Fair. Clearly there's work to be done on your diet. Take this quiz again in three months.

Less than 60 • Get a new start! Change your shopping habits, empty your cupboards and fridge, pay attention to what you order in restaurants! Follow the recommendations on pages 128–132, and take this quiz again in three months. If you're really worried about a low score, take your food record and this quiz to a nutrition professional for guidance.

Calibrating for Maximum Nutrition

If you scored low on a question, that's a signal that you need to zero in on that specific area and do some troubleshooting. Here are some commonsense suggestions on how to do just that.

Question 1 • Whole grain products provide B vitamins, vitamin E, and minerals like zinc, magnesium, and manganese. Enriched grain products can also provide iron. Eat at least six servings of unsweetened, low-fat grain products every day.

Questions 2 and 3 • Many women don't consume enough calcium, a mineral critical for bone health. Dairy products are the best sources. Other good sources include canned salmon (eaten with the bones) and tofu. (Four ounces of tofu have as much calcium as 4 ounces of milk.) Dark green leafy vegetables like broccoli and kale provide calcium, too. They also provide magnesium, folate, and vitamin B_6. At least three daily servings of calcium-rich foods can help ensure that women meet their Recommended Dietary Allowance. For men, two servings will do. (If you don't get that many, you may need to take a calcium supplement.)

Questions 4 and 6 • Your body can get vitamin A from compounds called carotenoids (including beta-carotene). Carotenoids are abundant in the orange-yellow vegetables and, to a lesser extent, in dark green leafy vegetables and some cruciferous vegetables. These vegetables may also offer cancer protection. Aim for one serving of orange-yellow and/or cruciferous vegetables every day, and at least one serving of dark green leafy vegetables a day.

Question 5 • Vitamin C is found in abundance in citrus fruits, other fruits (such as strawberries), and some vegetables (such as green peppers and broccoli). Try to eat one serving daily of vitamin C–rich foods.

Question 7 • Red meat can be high in fat, but it's an important source of easily absorbable iron, B vitamins, and other minerals, such as zinc. So lean red meat can be an important part of your diet. Chicken and turkey also contain these nutrients, although they have less iron than red meat. If you don't eat meat, make sure you're getting other iron-rich foods, such as grain products and dark green leafy vegetables. This is especially important for premenopausal women. Nonmeat sources of zinc include whole grains and shellfish.

Question 8 • Spreads, such as butter or hard margarine, can add unnecessary fat. Whenever possible, substitute fruit spreads or use nothing at all.

Question 9 • Although dairy products are good for your calcium intake, some can be high in fat. Choose low-fat or nonfat varieties.

Questions 10 and 11 • Processed meats tend to be high in fat. Choose home-cooked or canned water-packed meats or fish, which you've rinsed to reduce sodium. Always trim visible fats from meat and choose lean cuts.

Question 12 • Many processed chips, crackers, and cookies are loaded with fat. Try unbuttered popcorn, rice cakes or no-salt pretzels. For homemade treats, seek out low-fat recipes.

Question 13 • Say no to fried foods and greasy dressings. When eating out, order dressings and sauces on the side.

Question 14 • Oily salad dressing is high in fat. Try lemon juice or other delicious nonfat alternatives.

Questions 15 and 16 • Meat and cheese can be high in fat. Limit your intake to less than 6 ounces of meat daily and less than 2 ounces of full-fat cheeses.

Question 17 • Foods high in saturated fatty acids, like butter and hard margarine, can raise cholesterol levels. Softer margarines, like tub margarines, are lower in saturated fatty acids and higher in polyunsaturated fatty acids. Polyunsaturates, like corn and soy oil, can lower cholesterol. Monounsaturates, like olive oil and canola oil, can lower cholesterol, too. Experts recommend that your diet contain less than 30 percent of total calories from fat and that your total fat intake should be divided equally among the three kinds of fat.

Question 18 • Egg yolks, although an excellent source of nutrients, are high in cholesterol. If you're concerned about cholesterol, the American Heart Association recommends you limit intake to no more than two yolks a week.

Question 19 • Some processed foods are made with coconut or palm oil, which are high in saturated fatty acids. While it's not yet conclusive that these oils raise cholesterol as much as animal saturated fats, it's still prudent to read labels and steer away from them.

Questions 20 and 24 • To add more fiber to your daily diet, use products made with whole grains instead of products made with refined ingredients.

Question 21 • If cholesterol is a concern, aim for two oat servings a day (or other soluble fiber sources like apples or beans). *Note*: Most oat bran breads are not very high in oat bran! Oats or oat bran should be the first or second ingredient listed on the label.

Question 22 • Beans provide not only soluble fiber but also B vitamins and minerals; one serving a day is a good idea.

Question 23 • High-fiber breakfast cereals are a convenient source of fiber.

Question 25 • Whole fruits and vegetables are an important source of fiber. Many of them, like apples, contain high levels of both soluble and insoluble fiber.

Question 26 • Processed foods are often high in sodium. Read labels and look for low-sodium varieties or choose salt-free substitutes.

Question 27 • Even some sodium-reduced products can be high in sodium. Salt substitutes can also be high in sodium; check labels. Sometimes sodium is disguised: monosodium glutamate (MSG) is high in sodium. Break the habit of adding salt to your cooking, and remove the saltshaker from your table.

Question 28 • Alcohol not only adds extra calories with no nutrient payoff, but can deplete B vitamins and minerals and, in excess, damage the organs, add fat, and lead to liver disease. The National Research Council says alcohol offers no health benefits. Experts say that you should consume no more than 1 ounce of pure alcohol (about two beers) per day. And pregnant women shouldn't drink at all.

Question 29 • Sodas and sugary fruit drinks are high in calories, and low in nutrients. Drink fruit juices in moderation if you are watching your weight; they can be high in calories.

Question 30 • Too much caffeine can cause sleeplessness, and withdrawal triggers headaches in some people. There is a possible link between high consumption of regular coffee (more than five 6-ounce cups) and cardiovascular disease in men. Limit intake of all caffeine-containing beverages to no more than five servings a day.

Question 31 • Sweets provide few nutrients, a lot of calories and sugar, which cause cavities. They're often high in fat, too. Animal studies show that the combination of fat and sugar produces obesity.

Questions 32, 33, and 34 • Studies have shown that people who snack and eat irregularly have a harder time keeping their weight down. Limit snacking to twice a day.

The Sweet Truth about Your Sweet Tooth

By George L. Blackburn, M.D., Ph.D.

If nutritionists were to make out a report card on the American diet, the grades would be very puzzling indeed. There would be a lot of "A's" in the category of skim milk, fruits and vegetables, and leaner meats. In the last ten years Americans have significantly increased their consumption of these healthy, low-fat foods. But then there would be some lower marks. Researchers at the University of North Carolina School of Public Health recently analyzed data on the eating habits of thousands of American women, comparing the results of a diet survey taken in the mid-1970s with one taken in 1985. Along with the healthful changes noted above, they also found that women increased their consumption of high-fat desserts—like ice cream, cakes, cookies, pies, doughnuts, and granola bars—by about 6 percent between 1977 and 1985. What's going on here? Do Americans have a monumental sweet tooth, one so strong that it's overpowering our good sense about nutrition? And is this sweet tooth getting worse?

A Sweet Tooth—Or a "Fat Tooth"?

There's no doubt that sweets provide satisfaction, pleasure, oral gratification. But I'm not of the school that argues that the taste for sweets is a primal, genetic striving. Contrary to popular belief, breast milk does not have a sweet flavor.

Most people who think they have a sweet tooth really have a "fat tooth." That's a genetically and culturally determined desire for a certain amount of fat in their diet, which is driving them toward sweets. Think about it. The chocolate bar; the double-chocolate ice cream; the sugar-spiked yogurt; the chewy cookies. What draws you to them isn't just sweetness, it's the fat. If you read the label, the first ingredient might well be sugar, but close behind will be fat, and the percentage of calories from fat is probably well above the healthful 30 percent limit. (Calculate it yourself! Check the label on your processed sweets. Multiply fat grams per serving by nine and then divide the result by total calories per serving. That tells you the percent of calories from fat.)

Research shows that people with such an innate fat tooth have a programmed desire for a particular mix of carbohydrate, protein, and fat in their food. Every day, they'll try to eat to maintain a certain level of fat in the diet. When they grab a sweet, they're usually trying to achieve the level of fat that satisfies that deeper need.

Fat is not only the secret seducer in these desserts and snacks; it's also the villain. The fat increases our risk of heart disease and even certain kinds of cancer. Compared to that, sugar in moderation is relatively harmless, except to dental health (unless someone is a diabetic or has other special health problems).

How to Appease a Sweet Tooth

Yet many people still insist that they have a sweet tooth. And furthermore, they feel that if they don't get their sweets, they'll feel deprived.

If they won't settle for a banana or a nectarine, I offer advice that usually surprises them: "Fine. Then have your sugar straight up, without the fat." What does that mean? Toss the cheesecake and replace it with a light, low-fat, angel-food cake. Say No, thanks! to the afternoon doughnut and have a couple of plain low-fat gingersnaps instead. You'll have the sweets you desire, without unwanted side effects of fat.

Sweets and Weight Loss

Many people believe sweets are the culprit in obesity. That's another myth. If you have a sweet tooth and are overweight, it might well be a coincidence. The evidence: When researchers take sweets away from overweight people, they don't stop eating; they just overeat nonsweets, trying to satisfy their innate fat craving.

Losing weight is a complex undertaking, but it's important to put first things first. The most important tasks in weight loss are (1) to cut back on fat; (2) to eat complex carbohydrates, which are high in fiber; (3) to increase exercise; and (4) to reduce calories to a reasonable level (300 to 500 calories less than recommended intake for your height and weight). Dealing with a sweet craving is usually not a major task in weight loss, but it is one that can make a significant difference to maintaining weight loss.

If you can follow the "sugar straight up" rule and have your sugar in a nonfatty form, in moderate amounts, it should not impede weight loss. However, a few people find that sugar stimulates their appetite. If you find that eating sweets makes you hungrier, it's wiser to avoid them.

What about desserts and soft drinks sweetened with nonnutrient sweeteners like aspartame? Can they aid a weight-loss program? Research at our weight-loss clinic at the New England Deaconess Hospital indicates that nonnutrient sweeteners can make a small, positive difference to dieters. A study we conducted in 1988 (which, it should be noted, was supported by grants from the NutraSweet Company as well as the National Institutes of Health) looked at whether artificially sweetened foods and beverages affect weight loss.

Fifty-nine obese women and men (but mostly women) were put on a low-fat, calorie-reduced diet, about 1,000 calories a day for the women and 1,200 calories daily for the men. Emphasis was on low-fat foods, and there was also an exercise component and training in behavioral modification.

Half the people were encouraged to consume nonnutrient-sweetened foods—at least two daily—containing aspartame. They chose offerings like puddings, soft drinks, and frozen desserts. The other group was told to avoid use of all aspartame or saccharine-sweetened products, and were given food guides on low-calorie snacks and beverages free of nonnutrient sweeteners.

Both groups lost weight. After 12 weeks, the women who were permitted to eat nonnutrient sweeteners had lost 3.7 more pounds than women in the other group, a difference that is not statistically significant but does indicate that nonnutrient artificial sweeteners aren't a disadvantage to dieters, and might provide a small advantage.

It should be emphasized that both groups not only lost weight but enjoyed improvements in their health and quality of life. That's not because of sweets or lack of them; it's because they were on a balanced program with group support, behavioral training, exercise, and close monitoring.

I'd say the nonnutrient sweeteners provided a small additional advantage for two reasons. First, those sweeteners contain fewer calories than sugar. And second, the people eating the sweetened products may have felt less deprived and more satisfied because they could eat more desserts.

There has been great controversy over whether nonnutrient sweeteners are safe. They've been the subject of what are probably the most intensive Food and Drug Administration investigations of any food product. Since they've passed these tests, they don't pose a health threat.

My view is that there are other things the public should worry about, like fat in the diet, before they worry about the health impact of moderate amounts of nonnutrient sweeteners.

Is Margarine Better Than Butter?

Flip on the TV and you may notice the National Dairy Board is hitting its margarine-making foes with more than just a "little pat of butter"—a $14 million advertising smear campaign against its competition.

In short, the ads remind us that a little pat of sweet, creamy, and ever-so natural *real* butter has the same calories as an equal portion of its synthetic nemesis. Of course, it's all a friendly reminder to convince people to stick with butter and its better taste. There's no real intense mudslinging at margarine—this time. The Better Business Bureau banned those ads.

Not that butter people are the only ones spreading it on a bit thick. For decades, margarine has compared its taste (as well as its look, shape, smell, and sometimes even its package design) to that of butter. It seems to have worked. Charles Ehrhart, executive director of the National Association of Margarine Manufacturers, says several consumer groups and the American Heart Association have requested that margarine be substituted for butter in school lunch programs. Widespread institutional use of butter "gets kids hooked on butter early," says Ehrhart.

Apparently, few punches are pulled with America's toast on the line. Like the Hatfields and McCoys, the butter-versus-margarine feud has lasted generations—with no end in sight. For a long time, butter was winning: Until President Harry Truman signed the Margarine Act of 1950—which did away with taxes on margarine that were almost as much as its actual price—few people chose margarine. And with good reason: Besides the fact that margarine cost as much as butter (because of the taxes), a strong dairy lobby ensured that margarine had to be manufactured the color of "lard white" (except in a few states where it was allowed to be dyed pink). In those (before cholesterol awareness) days, the typical American ate about 10.5 pounds of butter and 5.8 pounds of margarine a year.

Margarine Takes the Lead

Now that's been reversed. U.S. Department of Agriculture statistics cited by Ehrhart show that in 1987, Americans averaged 10.5 pounds of margarine and 4.6 pounds of butter. And despite the nearly $14 million a year spent by the Dairy Board to convince people to stick with butter, Chuck Timpko, the board's manager of consumer research, notes that in 1988 in-home consumer use of butter dropped another 6 percent.

The reason: Besides being about half the cost, margarine is viewed as being "healthier." A tablespoon of butter has about 100 calories, 11 grams of fat (about 7 grams saturated and 4 unsaturated), and 30 milligrams of cholesterol. Margarine, manufactured from vegetable oils and artificially flavored and colored to look like butter, has no cholesterol and is low in saturated fats. (Of the 11 grams of fat in a tablespoon of margarine, usually 2 or 3 are saturated fat.)

But it's not a hands-down victory for margarine. "Margarine has no nutritional value—all you get is fat," says Robin Bagby, M.Ed., R.D., of the Penn State Nutrition Center. "The big misconception is that margarine has fewer calories. So people use it liberally. For people on a diet, you have to watch your *total* fat intake."

For those who believe margarine is just a manufactured collection of undesirable artery-clogging components, Michael Green, Ph.D., associate professor of nutrition science at the Pennsylvania State University, says that no study has conclusively linked any of margarine's fatty acids to negative outcomes. But he notes that "this concern has obviously led to the big increase in blends"—a combination of butter and margarine.

And the field is further crowded by what are called "spreads." To be called margarine, a product must by law be pretty much synthetic butter—it must be 80 percent fat, just like butter. But spreads can be just about anything they want, and what they tend to want to be is lower in saturated fat. So spreads have much higher percentages of pure veg-

COMPARING THE SPREADS

Product (1 Tbsp.)	Calories	Total Fat (g)	Polyunsaturated Fat (g)	Saturated Fat (g)	Cholesterol (mg)	Sodium (mg)	First Ingredient
Butter	100	11	4	7.1	31	140	Butterfat
Whipped butter	66	7	—	—	—	75	Butterfat
Butter-margarine blends	100	11	3	3	12	85–115	Varies
Margarine							
Stick	100	11	Varies	2	0	100	Varies
Tub	100	11	Varies	2	0	95	Varies
Whipped	66	7	Varies	1.3	0	80	Varies
Liquid	100	11	4–6	2	0	95–115	Liquid oil
Diet	50	6	2	1	0	110–140	Water
Spreads	50–75	6–7	2–3	1–1.5	0	60–110	Varies

SOURCE: National Association of Margarine Manufacturers.

etable oil—unhydrogenated—and thus even less saturated fat. They're also easier to spread—hence the name. In fact, there are even spreads in bottles now, but even Ehrhart admits that "most people aren't used to pouring spread on their toast."

Butter or margarine, spreads or blends? The bottom line: Moderate use of *all* of these products. For example, if you're worried about those weird fatty acids in margarine but you're worried about your cholesterol too, you can have butter—just not very much of it. Likewise, if you switch to margarine, you're not free of saturated fats: Eat 6 tablespoons of margarine and you may as well have had a couple of butter.

You can even make your own blends in a food processor (try 60 percent butter and 40 percent vegetable oil), as suggested by Dr. Green. So whether you favor your taste buds, your wallet, your arteries, your fear of the unknown, or any combination, there's a product on the shelves with your name on it. "If you're confused," says Bagby, "there's always jelly."

How to Get Your Fill of Fiber

By George L. Blackburn, M.D., Ph.D.

You're visiting a friend's house. She offers you a bowl of fudge ice cream and a large bran muffin. You're hungry, it's your favorite ice cream, but you're also trying to lose weight. What's the best thing you can do? (a) eat the muffin and refuse the ice cream; (b) scoop the ice cream on top of the muffin, hoping that what you read about fiber-subtracting calories from food is true; (c) refuse both, and ask your friend if she happens to have an apple and a glass of milk.

Answer: If you answered (a), you may have fallen into a common trap. Many "health" muffins boast about their fiber content, but are so high in calories and fat that they can do more harm than good.

If you said (b), sorry: Fiber doesn't carry huge numbers of calories out of the body. I'll explain that one shortly.

If you answered (c), you're right: Getting dietary fiber in the form of an apple (as part of a nutritionally balanced snack) really can help your weight-loss efforts. This combination will quell your appetite.

Who hasn't heard about the health benefits of fiber? This complex substance—the indigestible portion of whole grains, fruits, and vegetables—is important for everyone, not just people who need to lose weight. Fiber keeps the gastrointestinal tract functioning normally. A high-fiber diet can protect against and relieve constipation, intestinal disease, high cholesterol, diabetes, hemorrhoids, varicose veins, and ulcers. Scientists also hypothesize that it may ward off gallstones, colon cancer, and heart disease.

Although the government has not established a Recommended Dietary Allowance for fiber, all nutritional authorities agree we need a fiber-rich diet. Americans consume on average only about 11 to 15 grams a day; about 25 grams would be better, and I'd say an optimal diet should include about 35 grams per day.

The Stuff That Satisfies

A high-fiber eating plan is especially important for weight watchers, primarily because fiber satisfies the appetite. High-fiber foods must be chewed—and chewed and chewed. This allows more interaction with your taste buds so you have more sensory satisfaction.

The stomach's job is to turn entering solids into a form that's liquid enough to exit. Fibrous foods are an especially tough demolition job. It takes the stomach a long time to produce all the digestive juices, hormones, and enzymes to liquefy fibrous foods. So the stomach feels full longer and sends signals that say, "Don't send more! I'm not through digesting what you've eaten!" If you bring your fiber count up by increasing whole grains, fruits, and vegetables, you'll be less hungry for fattening foods. And you'll feel satisfied on fewer calories.

Vive la Différence

Since there are many different kinds of fiber, it's important to get fiber from many sources. Fiber falls into two basic categories: soluble and insoluble. They're both needed for good health and weight loss.

Soluble fiber is the kind that dissolves in water. Oat bran is the most famous form of soluble fiber, but it's also found in beans, barley, and some fruits and vegetables like squash, apples, citrus fruits, cauliflower, cabbage, strawberries, and potatoes. Soluble fiber slows the digestion of foods, so you're not hungry so soon. In large amounts, it can lower cholesterol and keep blood sugar levels steady. That's especially useful for dieters. On a low-fiber diet, your metabolism runs up peaks and down valleys, causing sudden energy losses and jittery feelings that can trigger bingeing. But soluble fiber helps keep your metabolism—and your appetite—on an even keel.

Insoluble fiber is the type found in whole wheat flour and bran, whole grains, vegetables, and in many fruits like apples and pears. It's a bulking agent, which means it prevents constipation. Constipation is common among dieters because they are eating less food. Not only is constipation uncomfortable, but at our weight-loss clinic at the New England Deaconess Hospital, we've found that less-constipated dieters have an easier time sticking to a weight-loss regimen.

How Fiber Won't Help

There's a rumor going around that you can lose weight on ice cream or candy bars, as long as you send them down the hatch with some bran or celery. The claim is that the fiber will escort a large portion of the calories out the back door. In fact, this is a wild exaggeration. On a low-fiber diet, an average stool may contain 100 calories, and if you eat more fiber, it will contain about 110 calories—an insignificant difference.

That's also why you should beware of baked goods, like certain commercial muffins that advertise that they're rich in fiber. A study of local oat bran muffins, conducted by the *New York Times* and the Center for Science in the Public Interest, uncovered one muffin bulging with 29 grams of fat (the equivalent of three single-serving bags of potato chips), and another weighing in at an incredible 824 calories! If your baked goods are packaged, read the labels and make sure the fiber count is over 3 grams per serving, and the fat and calorie count are modest.

A Fiber-Up Plan for Everyone

I've said that most Americans need to double their fiber intake, at least. But don't wake up tomorrow and pour bran meal into your breakfast bowl, eat a heaping dish of barley with mushrooms for lunch, and chow down a big plate of baked beans with broccoli for dinner, plus a couple of apples for snacks. The result of a sudden fiber increase is a day or two of stomach upset, gas, and diarrhea.

Instead, increase your fiber intake gradually. Most people who want to optimize the amount of fiber they eat should plan on taking three to nine months to reach their goal. (If you have irritable bowel syndrome, you'll need to stretch that even longer, under medical guidance. It could take two years.)

Your initial goal is to get to the point where you're at least meeting the National Research Council 1989 Diet and Health Report's "five/six" recommendation: five daily servings of fruits and vegetables and six daily servings of grains (meaning whole grain cereals, beans, cooked whole grains, breads, and pasta). This advice applies to everyone, not just weight watchers.

The bad news is that meeting the five/six goal might not get you up to 35 grams of fiber. The fiber content of different fruits, vegetables, and grains varies drastically.

So once you've met the five/six goal, the next step in your fiber-up program is to increase portion size and to focus on the highest-fiber foods (see "The 100 Best Fiber Foods" on page 143). Legumes (beans and peas) and fiber-

THE 100 BEST FIBER FOODS

Food	Portion	Dietary Fiber (g)
Bread		
Country oat	2 slices	6.0
Whole wheat, stone-ground	2 slices	4.5
Wheat, reduced-calorie	2 slices	4.0
Mixed grain	2 slices	3.2
Rye	2 slices	3.1
English muffin, wheat	1 muffin	3.0
Pita, whole wheat	1 pocket	2.8
Corn bread, whole ground	1 piece	2.7
Cracked wheat	2 slices	2.6
Bran muffin	1 muffin	2.5
Bran oat cakes	2 cakes	2.0
Breakfast Cereals, Cold		
100% bran-type		
With added fiber	$\frac{1}{2}$ cup	14.0
Regular	$\frac{1}{3}$ cup	10.0
With oat bran	$\frac{1}{2}$ cup	8.0
Multibran	$\frac{1}{3}$ cup	6.5
Oatmeal flakes	1 cup	6.0
Corn bran, ready-to-eat	$\frac{2}{3}$ cup	5.4
40% bran-type flakes	$\frac{2}{3}$ cup	5.3
Bran-type flakes with raisins	1 oz.	5.0
Oat bran, crunchy types	1 oz.	5.0
Bran squares	$\frac{2}{3}$ cup	4.6
Breakfast Cereals, Hot		
Multibran, creamy, instant, dry	$\frac{1}{4}$ cup	8.0
Oat bran	$\frac{1}{3}$ cup	5.0
Oatmeal, cooked	$\frac{3}{4}$ cup	1.6
Fruit		
Figs, dried	5	8.7
Pear	1 large	6.2
Blackberries	$\frac{1}{2}$ cup	4.5
Dates	5	3.2
Orange	1	3.1
Raspberries	$\frac{1}{2}$ cup	3.1
Prunes	5	3.0
Apple, with skin	1	3.0
Strawberries	$\frac{3}{4}$ cup	2.9
Apricots, dried	10 halves	2.7
Kiwi	1	2.6
Nectarine	1	2.2
Cantaloupe	$\frac{1}{2}$	2.0
Raisins	$\frac{1}{4}$	1.9
Banana	1	1.8
Plums	3 small	1.8
Blueberries	$\frac{1}{2}$ cup	1.7
Apricots	2	1.5

(continued)

THE 100 BEST FIBER FOODS—*Continued*

Food	Portion	Dietary Fiber (g)
Grains		
Corn bran, raw	1 oz.	23.0
Wheat bran, toasted	1 oz.	14.1
Rice bran, raw	1 oz.	6.2–9.5
Bulgur, raw	1 oz.	5.2
Barley, raw	1 oz.	4.9
Oat bran, raw	1 oz.	4.5
Wheat flour, whole grain	1 oz.	3.6
Cornmeal, whole grain	1 oz.	3.1
Wheat germ	1 oz.	3.0
Oats, rolled, dry	1 oz.	2.9
Millet, hulled, raw	1 oz.	2.4
Legumes		
Baked beans, vegetarian, canned	½ cup	9.8
Kidney, cooked	½ cup	9.0
Pintos, cooked	½ cup	8.9
Black-eyed peas, cooked	½ cup	8.3
Miso (soybeans)	½ cup	7.5
Chick-peas	½ cup	7.0
Limas, cooked	½ cup	6.8
Navy, cooked	½ cup	6.8
Lentils, cooked	½ cup	5.2
White, cooked	½ cup	5.0
Green peas, cooked	½ cup	2.4
Nuts and Seeds		
Almonds, oil-roasted	¼ cup	4.4
Pistachio nuts	¼ cup	3.5
Mixed nuts, oil-roasted	¼ cup	3.2
Peanuts	¼ cup	3.2
Pecans	¼ cup	2.3
Rice, Pasta, and Tortillas		
Pasta, multigrain		
With quinoa, dry	2 oz.	8.0
With triticale, dry	2 oz.	6.5
With oat bran, dry	2 oz.	6.0
Whole wheat, dry	2 oz.	6.0
Rice		
Wild, cooked	½ cup	5.3
Brown, long-grain, cooked	½ cup	1.7
Tortilla, corn	2 shells	3.1
Snacks		
Cookies		
Graham crackers, oat bran	1.2 oz.	3.0
Oat plus fruit	2	3.0
Oat bran	2	2.8
Fig bars	2	1.3

Food	Portion	Dietary Fiber (g)
Crackers		
Stone-ground	1 oz.	3.9
Crisps, thin oat	½ oz.	3.2
Crisps, thin rye	½ oz.	3.0
Hearty wheat	4	3.0
Whole wheat saltines	5	1.0
Popcorn, gourmet	½ oz.	2.0
Vegetables		
Artichokes, raw	1 med.	6.7
Brussels sprouts, boiled	5	4.5
Mixed, frozen, cooked	½ cup	3.5
Sweet potato, baked	1	3.4
Corn, cooked	1 ear	2.8
Parsley, chopped	1 cup	2.8
Parsnips, cooked	½ cup	2.7
Broccoli, raw, chopped	1 cup	2.5
Potato, with skin	1 med.	2.5
Carrots, raw	1	2.3
Turnip greens, boiled	½ cup	2.2
Spinach, boiled	½ cup	2.1
Asparagus, cut	1 cup	2.0
Cauliflower, cooked	5 florets	2.0
Zucchini, cooked	½ cup	1.8
Cabbage, raw, shredded	1 cup	1.7
Green beans, string, cooked	½ cup	1.6
Tomato, raw	1 med.	1.5

SOURCES: Adapted from "Soluble and Total Dietary Fiber in Selected Foods," and "Provisional Table on the Dietary Fiber Content of Selected Foods," USDA Human Nutrition Information Service.

Fiber Facts (Chicago: The American Dietetic Association, 1986). Reprinted in "Dietary Fiber and Health," *Journal of the American Medical Association,* July 1989.

"Dietary Fiber Content of Selected Foods," *American Journal of Clinical Nutrition,* 1988.

Plant Fiber in Foods, James W. Anderson (HCF Nutrition Research Foundation, Inc., 1986).

NOTE: Top sources of soluble fiber include oat and barley products, legumes, and fruit.

rich fruits like apples, prunes, raspberries, and pears are especially good choices.

People who are actively losing weight should make a special effort to select the highest fiber foods. Sometimes that's easier said than done. For example, if you're deciding between a large salad and small baked potato, or a small salad and a large baked potato, which would you choose? Go for the big potato. Lettuce isn't a terrific source of fiber—it's 90 percent water—while the potato will really fill you up. (Any time you're losing weight, take a daily multivitamin supplement. Don't let your weight-loss phase last for more than 12 weeks. Then try to maintain that loss for at least three months before trying to lose any more weight.)

What about Fiber Supplements?

Fiber supplements, in the form of pills and powders, are popular weight-loss aids, but like most nutritionists I'm not enthusiastic about them. Improper use of fiber supplements can lead to serious fiber overdoses that can create obstructions in the colon.

Some of these supplements are so low in fiber, containing as little as $\frac{1}{2}$ gram per tablet, that they're virtually useless. Any product that claims to be high in fiber, whether it's a supplement, a cereal, or a whole grain bread, should contain at least 3 grams of fiber per serving.

And finally, the biggest problem with fiber supplements is that they're a crutch, part of an eating style that can't be sustained. For successful weight loss and maintenance, and for good health, you have to develop a satisfying way of eating that will last a lifetime. That's why it's important to get your fiber from many sources.

Cheese Can Be Heart Healthy

By Judith Benn Hurley,
with the Rodale Food Center

Like a hefty wedge of Swiss, the argument that cheese is a healthy food has some holes in it. Sure, a 1-ounce slice can go a long way to satisfy your daily protein requirement. And cheese is an excellent source of calcium. Unfortunately, many cheeses contain upward of 70 percent fat. That may sound disheartening for those of you watching your weight or cholesterol. But before you throw out the lasagna with the mozzarella, consider this: Cheesemakers are responding to consumer demand for lower-fat products, so lighter types are available. A quick scan of supermarket shelves will identify suitable brands.

Remember, too, there are many types of cheese. The very soft kinds, such as cottage cheese, fromage blanc, and yogurt cheese, tend to be the leanest. Choose low-fat and dry-curd versions of cottage cheese for everyday cooking. Make your own cream cheese substitute from nonfat yogurt (see "Amazing Yogurt Cheese" on page 148).

You can easily prepare fromage blanc, a silky, nonfat sour cream substitute, using skim milk and a starter culture available from the New England Cheesemaking Supply Company, 85 Main St., Ashfield, MA 01330; call (413) 628-3808.

Prices are $5.95 (postpaid) for five packets of culture or $12.95 (plus $3 postage and handling) for a starter kit consisting of cheesecloth, a dairy thermometer, four packets of starter culture, and a recipe book. Detailed directions for making fromage blanc are included.

Some very hard cheeses can be grated and used sparingly to enliven the taste of other foods. A tablespoon of grated Parmesan, for example, costs less than 2 grams of fat and gives a plate of pasta just the right amount of oomph—without unbalancing its excellent fat ratio. A tablespoon of grated sapsago, a very tasty low-fat cheese similar in texture to Parmesan, has a mere trace of fat.

On occasions when you want a cheese meal—say, a cheese sandwich—choose a reduced-fat variety and team it up with other high-carbohydrate, low-fat foods. Surround 1 ounce of reduced-fat Cheddar, for example, with two slices of whole grain bread spread with a little mustard (hold the mayo). Serve with baked beans, an apple, and skim milk. Your meal now has only 24 percent of calories from fat.

For those counting every milligram of cholesterol, there are no-cholesterol soy-based cheeses on the market. And for those concerned about sodium, there are low-sodium varieties. Again, read labels. That way you can satisfy the cheese lover in you without sabotaging your health.

Amazing Yogurt Cheese

What's lusciously smooth and creamy, with only a fraction of cream cheese's calories and none of its fat? Yogurt cheese. And it's a snap to make at home.

Just line a large strainer with either cheesecloth, white paper towels, or a coffee filter. (Or use a special yogurt-cheese funnel.) Spoon in 4 cups of plain nonfat yogurt, refrigerate and let drain overnight. You'll end up with $1\frac{1}{2}$ to 2 cups of nonfat yogurt cheese. Store your cheese covered in the refrigerator.

Each $\frac{1}{4}$-cup portion (2 ounces) has about 34 calories and no fat—compared with 198 calories and over 19 grams of fat for cream cheese.

Note: Some brands of yogurt have emulsifiers or stabilizers in them that prevent the whey from draining off. Reading the label isn't always enough to tell you whether a particular yogurt is drainable. So try this test at home: Take a big spoonful of yogurt out of the container, leaving a depression. If the hole starts to fill with liquid within 10 minutes, you should have success making yogurt cheese from this particular brand.

Here are some ways to use your yogurt cheese:

• Fold in chives and use to top baked potatoes or potato skins.
• Add fresh or dried herbs and use as a savory spread for toast or crackers.
• Mix with minced smoked turkey and use in place of cream cheese on bagels.
• Stir in orange juice concentrate and minced fruit (such as strawberries). Use as a topping for muffins, pancakes, or waffles.
• Add homemade pesto or salsa and use as a dip for crisp raw vegetables.

Elbows and Cheese

1½ cups uncooked elbow macaroni

⅔ cup shredded soy Cheddar

½ cup dry-curd cottage cheese

½ cup skim milk

2 teaspoons Dijon mustard

2 egg whites

   hot pepper sauce, to taste

1 slice whole wheat bread

Cook the macaroni in a large pot of boiling water until not quite tender, about 8 minutes. Drain.

Coat a 1-quart casserole dish with nonstick spray. Add macaroni and Cheddar. Toss to combine.

In a blender, purée the cottage cheese, milk, 1 teaspoon mustard, egg whites, and hot pepper sauce. Pour over the macaroni and stir lightly to distribute.

Tear the bread into pieces and place in a food processor with the remaining mustard. Process into fine crumbs. Sprinkle over the casserole.

Bake at 350°F for 40 minutes.

Makes 4 servings (264 calories, 5.1 grams fat [18% of calories], 15.2 grams protein, 2 milligrams cholesterol, 229 milligrams sodium per serving)

Cheese-Stuffed Blintzes

This recipe uses fromage blanc, which requires a starter culture. See page 147 for ordering information.

Blintzes

6 ounces whole wheat pastry flour (about ⅓ cup)

½ teaspoon baking powder

1 egg white

⅔ cup skim milk

Filling

1 cup fromage blanc

2 tablespoons honey

¼ teaspoon ground cinnamon

Garnish

blueberries, cooked pears, or applesauce

grated orange or lemon rind

To make the blintzes: In a medium bowl, whisk together the flour and baking powder. Whisk in the egg white and milk. Continue whisking until free of lumps.

Coat a small nonstick frying pan with nonstick spray. Place the pan over medium-high heat. Pour in about 3 tablespoons of batter and swirl it around to coat the bottom of the pan.

Cook the blintz for about 1 minute, until the top is dry and the bottom is lightly browned. Flip the blintz out onto a rack or tea towel by turning the pan upside down. Continue making blintzes with the remaining batter.

To make the filling: In a small bowl, mix the fromage blanc, honey, and cinnamon.

To fill the blintzes, lay each blintz on a counter. Spoon a rounded tablespoon of the filling onto the middle of the blintz. Fold the bottom of the blintz over the cheese. Then fold in the sides. Finish by rolling the whole thing up into a little pouch.

Coat a large nonstick frying pan with nonstick spray. Heat over medium heat. Add the blintzes and cook for a few minutes on each side to lightly brown.

Serve garnished with blueberries, pears, or applesauce and orange or lemon rind.

Makes 8 (115 calories, 0.9 gram fat [7% of calories], 2.7 grams dietary fiber, 5.3 grams protein, 2 milligrams cholesterol, 59 milligrams sodium per blintz. Also a good source of thiamine, phosphorus, and magnesium)

Marinated Cheese Buttons

1 tablespoon red wine vinegar
2 tablespoons chicken stock
1 teaspoon canola oil
1 teaspoon dried oregano
1 teaspoon dried basil or thyme
1 teaspoon coarse mustard
  freshly ground black pepper, to taste
½ cup nonfat yogurt cheese
6 slices French bread, halved

In a 9-inch glass pie plate, whisk together the vinegar, stock, oil, oregano, basil or thyme, mustard, and pepper.

Roll well-rounded teaspoons of the yogurt cheese between your hands to form smooth balls. If the balls become sticky, wet your hands a bit with the marinade. Flatten the balls slightly and place in the marinade. Use a spoon to drizzle marinade over them.

Cover the dish and refrigerate for 30 minutes. Serve slightly chilled or at room temperature on pieces of bread.

Makes 12 (64 calories, 1.1 grams fat [16% of calories], 2.5 grams protein, 0 milligrams cholesterol, 103 milligrams sodium per button)

Cheese-Stuffed Potatoes

2 large potatoes, baked
⅓ cup dry-curd cottage cheese
3 tablespoons buttermilk
1 small carrot, grated
1 tablespoon minced fresh parsley
½ teaspoon dried thyme
  pinch of ground paprika
1 tablespoon grated Parmesan cheese

Slice the potatoes in half lengthwise. Scoop out the centers with a spoon, leaving ¼-inch shells.

In a medium bowl, mash the potato flesh roughly with a fork. Add the cottage cheese, buttermilk, carrot, parsley, thyme, and paprika. Mix well.

Spoon the filling into the shells. Sprinkle with the Parmesan.

Place the potatoes on a broiler pan and broil until lightly browned and warmed through, about 4 to 5 minutes.

Makes 4 servings (86 calories, 0.8 gram fat [8% of calories], 5 grams protein, 2 milligrams cholesterol, 55 milligrams sodium per serving. Also a good source of vitamins A and C)

Shells with Spring Vegetables and Cheese

⅔ cup dry-curd cottage cheese

¼ cup snipped chives

1 leek, minced

2 scallions, minced

2 cloves garlic, minced

1 carrot, grated

1 teaspoon Dijon mustard

½ teaspoon dried tarragon

1 egg white

¼ teaspoon black pepper

12 large pasta shells, cooked

⅔ cup tomato sauce

1 tablespoon grated Parmesan cheese

In a medium bowl, combine the cottage cheese, chives, leeks, scallions, garlic, carrot, mustard, tarragon, egg white, and pepper.

Use a spoon to stuff the filling into the shells.

Spread most of the tomato sauce in the bottom of a 9 × 9-inch baking dish. Add the shells. Drizzle with the remaining sauce. Sprinkle with the Parmesan.

Cover the dish with a lid or foil. Bake at 350°F for 20 to 30 minutes, or until the filling has set. Serve warm or at room temperature.

Makes 4 servings (187 calories, 2.6 grams fat [12% of calories], 1 gram dietary fiber, 10.6 grams protein, 3 milligrams cholesterol, 317 milligrams sodium per serving. Also a good source of thiamine)

Green-Chili and Cheese Rolls

½ pound mushrooms, coarsely chopped

3 scallions, chopped

3 mild green chili peppers, minced

2 cloves garlic, minced

½ teaspoon dried basil

1 tablespoon dry-curd cottage cheese

1 tablespoon nonfat yogurt cheese

1 tablespoon soy mozzarella or part-skim mozzarella

15 square wonton skins

½ teaspoon oil

Mince the mushrooms and scallions in a food processor. Place in a large nonstick frying pan with the chilies, garlic, and basil. Cook over medium-high heat until all the liquid evaporates, about 4 minutes. Let cool.

Stir the cottage cheese, yogurt cheese, and mozzarella into the mushroom mixture.

To assemble each roll, set a wonton skin flat on the counter with a corner pointed toward you. Lightly wet the outer edges of the skin with water. Place about 2 teaspoons of the filling just below the center of the skin. Fold the point that's toward you over the filling. Press down the edges around the filling. Fold in the left and right corners and roll up to finish. Place the rolls on a cake rack set on a baking sheet.

Very lightly coat the top of each roll with vegetable oil (use your finger). Place the baking sheet in the oven and bake the rolls at 450°F for 7 minutes, or until they turn light brown. Flip the rolls and coat with a bit more oil. Bake another 7 minutes.

Makes 15 (30 calories, 0.7 gram fat [21% of calories], 1.1 grams protein, 0 milligrams cholesterol, 3 milligrams sodium per roll)

A SENSIBLE GUIDE TO CHEESE SELECTION

Cheese/ Portion	Calories	Cholesterol (mg)	Fat (g)	Calories from Fat (%)
Cheddar, light, 1 oz.	80	20	5	56
Colby, low-fat, 1 oz.	85	20	5	53
Cottage, ½ cup				
Dry-curd	62	5	0.3	5
1% low-fat	82	5	1.2	13
2% low-fat	102	10	2.2	19
Edam, reduced-fat, 1 oz.	65	NA	3.1	43
Farmer, 1 oz.	81	18	5	56
Fromage blanc, 1 oz.	18	1.2	0.5	Trace
Gammelost, 1 oz.	56	3	Trace	0
Monterey Jack, low-fat, 1 oz.	80	15	5	56
Mozzarella, part-skim, 1 oz.	72	16	4.5	56
Parmesan, grated, 1 Tbsp.	23	4	1.9	59
Ricotta, light, 1 oz.	40	7	2	45
Sapsago, grated, 1 Tbsp.	12	1.6	0.4	26
Yogurt cheese, non-fat, 1 oz.	17	0.3	0	0

NOTE: Nutrition information label should be checked for product variation among manufacturers.

Tools for Low-Fat Cooking

How healthy is your kitchen? If traditional frying pans, deep fryers, or butter molds still take up space in your kitchen cabinets, it's not in top form. And in all probability, neither are you.

The right cookware can bring both you and your kitchen up to snuff. Utensils that help cut fat, calories, and cholesterol can make cooking a healthy joy. They let you start with the leanest, lowest-calorie foods and turn them into luscious repasts. Here are some items you'll probably find indispensable for cholesterol-lowering cookery, and at the end of the chapter are some tasty low-fat recipes to try.

Vertical Poultry Roaster • It's the ultimate in effortless low-fat cooking. Just slide a chicken onto one of these roasters, and watch the fat drip away as the bird cooks. That means your chicken—or Cornish hen, turkey, duck, capon, or goose—doesn't sit in a pool of grease as it roasts. In addition, the roaster holds poultry upright so air can circulate around it, leaving the meat moist and evenly cooked without the need for basting with butter or other high-calorie fats.

Make fabulous salads and sandwiches by roasting a chicken and refrigerating it until needed. Always remove the skin for tasty, low-fat dining. A bonus for the busy: Poultry cooks faster on a vertical roaster than by regular roasting methods. Available for about $17 from the Wooden Spoon Catalog; call (800) 431-2207 or in Connecticut (203) 664-0303 for more information.

Glass Food Steamer • How can a glass steamer help you cut fat more than another type of steamer? By allowing you to feast with your eyes: If you're able to watch that crisp emerald-green broccoli or those vibrant carrots as they cook, you simply won't allow them to become limp and mushy. And crisp, succulent veggies just beg to be enjoyed *au naturel* or with freshly ground pepper or minced herbs. You won't even think about dousing them with butter or a fatty sauce. Available for about $28 from the Wooden Spoon Catalog.

Gentle Cooker • The new generation of pressure cookers is safer, better looking, and easier to use. Now you can prepare cholesterol-fighting beans and brown rice in a fraction of the time required by normal methods. Unsoaked black beans take only 35 minutes. Low-fat vegetable soups can be ready in about 15 minutes—but their flavors are nicely developed as though they've undergone long simmering. Even lean meats, which often become tough when cooked without added fat, emerge tender and juicy from a pressure cooker. Available for about $70 from the Wooden Spoon Catalog.

Soft-Serve Frozen-Dessert Machine • The biggest complaint about homemade fat-free, sugar-free frozen desserts is that they become hard as rocks in the freezer. A soft-serve machine turns those rocks into creamy, cholesterol-free treats. You can process frozen fruits (like strawberries, blueberries, and bananas) into creamy, silky sensations. Try all three flavors for a skinny parfait. Available for about $70 from the Chef's Catalog; call (800) 338-3232 for more information.

Electric Spice Grinder • A spice grinder finely minces or purées herbs and spices into highly aromatic, cholesterol-free flavorings for use in sauces, dressings, marinades, soups, and stews.

A spice grinder differs from a pepper mill in that it can handle fresh, leafy herbs and garlic cloves or pieces of ginger without clogging. You can also purée a combination of dry and moist flavorings. Start with the moist first (try shallot and fresh oregano), then add dried aromatics (such as cumin seed and coriander seed). Available for about $35 in department stores and gourmet cookware shops.

Nonstick Frying Pan • No doubt you're already familiar with this indispensable member of the low-fat arsenal. But are you frustrated by pans that scratch at the drop of a spatula—no matter how careful you are? Well, rejoice! There's a new generation of nonstick cookware that doesn't have to be pampered or discarded regularly. SilverStone II pans are darker and smoother than ever. Better yet, they're available in a heavier, professional weight to ensure even cooking. Many foods, like spinach and chopped onion, virtually glide over the surface without a drop of fat. SilverStone skillets available from $30 in department stores.

Yogurt-Cheese Maker • It's a snap to make nonfat yogurt cheese with this reusable funnel. Simply spoon 2 cups of nonfat yogurt into the funnel and let it drain overnight (loosely covered and refrigerated). In the morning you'll have about ¾ cup of creamy nonfat spread.

Flavor it with chopped pineapple and raisins as a topping for warm oat-bran muffins. Or stir in thyme and prepared mustard as a fat-free dressing for turkey sandwiches. With the addition of minced shallots and your favorite herb (try rosemary), you've got a tasty dip for vegetables. Store yogurt cheese covered in the refrigerator, where it will keep for about a week. Available for about $10 from the Wooden Spoon Catalog.

Knife Sharpener • Get the low-fat edge with a sharp knife. Trimming every last speck of fat from meats is so much easier with sharp cutlery. Ditto for removing skin from poultry and slicing up mounds of luscious low-fat vegetables. Available for about $20 in department stores and gourmet cookware shops.

Cast-Iron Cookware • Cast iron is the original nonstick cookware. Well-seasoned cast iron leaves foods naturally juicy without added fat. And nowadays some cast iron comes preseasoned, so you can use it right away. Heavy-bottomed frying pans sear delicate foods (like scallops) gently without a drop of fat. And stovetop grillpans have nifty ridges that allow any fat in burgers to drain out of harm's way. (Note that even preseasoned cast iron needs to be used a few times before it's ready for serious cooking. Be sure to follow the manufacturer's instructions.) Available in department stores and gourmet cookware shops. From $20 for a 12-inch skillet; about $40 for a grillpan.

Citrus Reamer • Operating on the same principle as an old-fashioned orange juicer, the reamer gives you flavorful (and cholesterol-lowering) pulp as well as juice. So lemon, orange, lime, and tangerine juices just burst with fat-free zip. Use the aromatic juice and pulp to spice up marinades, beverages, soups, salad dressings, and frozen desserts.

Reamers come in wood, plastic, and electric models. Available from $3 in most department stores.

Marinated Roast Chicken

2 cloves garlic, peeled

¼ cup chopped parsley

1 tablespoon Dijon mustard

1 teaspoon red pepper flakes

1 teaspoon fennel or dill seeds

2 lemons, halved

1 roasting chicken (4 to 5 pounds)

Grind the garlic, parsley, and mustard in an electric spice grinder until very finely minced. Add the pepper flakes and fennel or dill. Process until the seeds are very finely minced. (You may also do this by hand with a mortar and pestle; add the ingredients in the same order.)

Use a citrus reamer to extract the juice and pulp from the lemons. If your spice grinder is large enough, pour in the juice and process into a thin paste. (Otherwise, transfer spices to a small bowl and whisk in the juice.)

Rub the marinade all over the chicken. Let stand, refrigerated, for 2 hours (or overnight, if desired).

Remove enough racks from your oven so there will be enough room to stand the chicken upright. Preheat oven to 450°F.

Set a vertical roaster in a roasting pan. Pour about 1 inch of water into the pan. Place the chicken on the vertical roaster. Carefully set the roasting pan on either the lowest rack or directly on the floor of the oven.

Immediately reduce the oven temperature to 350°F. Roast for 16 to 17 minutes per pound or until a thermometer inserted in a thigh registers 190°F.

Let the chicken stand for about 10 minutes before carving. Remove the skin before eating.

Makes 4 servings (415 calories, 4.7 grams fat [11% of calories], 0.3 gram dietary fiber, 83.9 grams protein, 210 milligrams cholesterol, 292 milligrams sodium per serving. Also a good source of riboflavin, niacin, and vitamin B_6)

Potato Crisps

8 small potatoes (about ¾ pound)
2 teaspoons olive oil or canola oil
½ teaspoon dried oregano

Slice the potatoes into ¼-inch disks. Then arrange them in a 9-inch glass pie plate. Add 1 tablespoon of water. Cover with vented plastic wrap and microwave on high (100 percent) until just tender, about 3 minutes. (If you don't have a microwave, blanch the potatoes in boiling water for 4 or 5 minutes.)

Pat the potatoes dry. Toss with the oil and oregano.

Heat a well-seasoned cast-iron frying pan on high heat for 2 minutes. Add the potatoes and sizzle on medium-high heat until mottled with brown and very slightly puffed, about 12 to 14 minutes on each side. Be sure to flip them several times during cooking. Serve warm.

Makes 4 servings (83 calories, 2.4 grams fat [25% of calories], 2.4 grams dietary fiber, 1.9 grams protein, 0 milligrams cholesterol, 6 milligrams sodium per serving)

Stovetop-Grilled Swordfish

Potato Crisps (see recipe above)
1 pound swordfish
2 teaspoons light mayonnaise
½ teaspoon dillweed

Prepare Potato Crisps according to recipe. About 15 minutes before crisps are finished cooking, start preparing fish.

Cut fish into ½-inch-thick slices. Rub with the light mayonnaise and sprinkle with the dill.

Preheat a cast-iron grillpan on high for 5 minutes. Add the fish and reduce the heat to medium-high. Let the fish sizzle for about 45 seconds, then flip so grill marks appear on both sides. Continue to sizzle the fish until cooked through, about 5 minutes. Serve with the potatoes.

Makes 4 servings (205 calories, 6.6 grams fat [29% of calories], 2.3 grams dietary fiber, 21.2 grams protein, 38 milligrams cholesterol, 102 milligrams sodium per serving. Also a good source of niacin and vitamin B_{12})

Frozen Pineapple-Banana Yogurt

1¼ cups pineapple chunks (about ½ pound)

1 medium banana, peeled

2 tablespoons maple syrup (optional)

2 cups plain nonfat yogurt

Purée the pineapple and banana in a food processor. If the fruit needs sweetening, add the maple syrup. Stir in the yogurt.

Spoon the mixture into two ice-cube trays. Freeze until solid. When frozen, pop the cubes out of the trays and store in a plastic bag.

When you're ready for yogurt, process as many cubes as needed in the soft-serve machine according to the manufacturer's directions.

Makes 5 to 6 servings (94 calories, 0.5 gram fat [4% of calories], 1.2 grams dietary fiber, 5.6 grams protein, 2 milligrams cholesterol, 70 milligrams sodium per serving. Also a good source of riboflavin and calcium)

NOTE: Some soft-serve frozen-dessert machines function as ice-cream makers. If yours does, pour the yogurt mixture into the machine and process the dessert according to the manufacturer's directions.

Nutrition Nuggets: Surprising Health Facts about Food

No, all nuts are not created equal. Candy-coated snacks aren't necessarily disastrous nutritional choices. And—surprise!—milk labeled "low-fat" can contain more butterfat than buttermilk.

Confused? Don't be. Just take your reading glasses to the grocery store (so you won't miss the fine print on the labels). And take a gander at the following food facts—because most of the time, you just can't judge the health value of a food by its label, looks, or reputation. You simply have to know.

- Roasted chestnuts make great diet snacks, with less than 5 percent of their calories from fat.
- Macadamia nuts, on the other hand, deliver 95 percent of calories in fat—albeit most is monounsaturated.
- Oil-popped popcorn can be 45 percent fat, even if it's not buttered!
- Caramel-coated popcorn (usually air-popped) gets only 7 percent of its calories from fat.
- Spinach is considered a good source of iron, but less than 2 percent of it is bioavailable; that means up to 98 percent of the iron in the plant cannot be readily absorbed by the body.
- By drinking orange juice with your meals, you can boost your body's absorption of iron from plant foods by as much as 400 percent, because vitamin C, which is abundant in oranges, enhances iron's bioavailability.
- Red peppers have almost 1½ times more vitamin C than green—and almost 11 times as many carotenoids, which your body converts to vitamin A.
- Chasing an iron-rich dinner with a cup of coffee or tea can reduce your body's absorption of the mineral by 40 to 85 percent. The culprit, apparently, is the tannin in tea and coffee, which binds iron.

- In terms of vitamin C content, oranges pale in comparison to black currants. One-half cup of black currants has almost $1\frac{1}{2}$ times the vitamin C of an orange.
- Ounce for ounce, cauliflower also has more vitamin C than oranges. In fact, just 1 cup of cauliflower delivers more than your daily requirement.
- Pink or ruby red grapefruit contains up to 26 times more carotenoids (including beta-carotene) than the white variety.
- Tofu, a high-protein soybean curd, actually contains more than half of its calories in fat. The good news is that, unlike animal protein, which can be high in saturated fat and cholesterol, tofu is mostly monounsaturated and polyunsaturated fat with no cholesterol.
- Not all pork products are as fatty as you might think; lean pork tenderloin gets only 26 percent of its calories from fat.
- Not all turkey products are as lean as you might think. While skinless turkey breast has less than 5 percent fat calories, turkey bologna and franks can contain up to 70 percent of their calories in fat.
- A $3\frac{1}{2}$-ounce serving of roast venison has fewer calories and fewer calories from fat than roasted skinless chicken breast.
- Trimming visible fat from meat and skinning poultry can cut the saturated fat content by more than one-half; interestingly, however, it has very little effect on the cholesterol content.
- Shellfish are generally high in cholesterol but surprisingly low in saturated fat; four large raw shrimp, for example, tip the scale with 152 milligrams of cholesterol but a scant $\frac{1}{3}$ of a gram of saturated fat.
- Even though it sounds rich, buttermilk has less fat per serving than 1 percent low-fat milk.
- Two percent low-fat milk is 2 percent fat by weight, but actually contains 35 percent of calories from fat; 1 percent low-fat milk is about 23 percent fat calories.
- Less than 5 percent of the calories in skim milk come from fat.

• An ounce of fudge has about half the fat of a 1-ounce brownie.

• Cocoa reduces symptoms of lactose intolerance. That means some of the people who are lactose intolerant can drink chocolate milk with fewer unpleasant symptoms, such as bloating and cramping.

• The cocoa in chocolate milk does not bind calcium, as once thought, so you can enjoy your chocolate treat and still reap the full benefit of the calcium.

• It's not true that all the alcohol used in cooking evaporates. In tests sponsored by the U.S. Department of Agriculture, 5 to 85 percent of the alcohol was retained in food after heating.

• Canola oil contains a kind of fatty acid that's converted in the body to eicosapentaenoic acid (EPA), which is a type of health-promoting fat abundant in certain fish oils.

• Ounce for ounce, cranberries have twice as much total dietary fiber as apples—and black currants contain four times as much.

• Tabbouleh contains three times as much fiber per serving as a tossed green salad.

• Cooked brussels sprouts, corn, zucchini, pintos, lima beans, raw cauliflower, and fresh currants all have as much cholesterol-lowering soluble fiber per $\frac{1}{2}$ cup as does cooked oatmeal.

• Ounce for ounce, kale contains more bioavailable calcium than the calcium champ itself, milk.

• A potato has almost double the potassium of a banana.

Catch On to the New Wave of Seafood Cooking

You might say there's something fishy going on in America. From sea to shining sea, people are catching on to the health benefits of fish and other seafoods, those heart-healthy gems of the ocean. Once touted as brain food, fish is perhaps one of the smartest choices you can make. It's lower in fat than most meats and high in important nutrients like magnesium, potassium, zinc, and iron. And most types—including shellfish—are fine sources of omega-3 fatty acids, those super dietary compounds that seem to buoy up heart health.

But hold the boat. Aren't shellfish awash with cholesterol, a leading contributor to heart disease? Although lobster and shrimp do contain more cholesterol than meat and poultry, levels for clams, oysters, and scallops are lower than formerly thought, and they can be eaten two or three times a week. All shellfish—including shrimp and lobster—are low in saturated fat, the main villain in heart disease. The American Heart Association now says that one serving of shrimp or lobster a week is perfectly acceptable for people on a prudent (low-fat, low-cholesterol) diet.

As for finned fish, nutrition experts recommend at least two servings a week, and the more the merrier. But if you're like a fish out of water when it comes to seafood cookery, take heart.

Prevention went from coast to coast for the best tips, techniques, and recipes from three top regional seafood chefs. With their help you'll see just how easy it is to prepare fish at home. And here's a promise: Once you've mastered the art of seafood cookery, you'll never have to fish for compliments again!

Chef Roland Czekelius, Chatham Bars Inn, Chatham, Massachusetts

The bounty of fresh seafood around Cape Cod inspires chef Roland Czekelius to create hearty yet heart-healthy food at the Chatham Bars Inn. Having the Atlantic Ocean at his kitchen door makes it easy for him to serve up light, low-fat seafood dishes featuring cod, haddock, clams, scallops, and other seafoods that are rich in omega-3's. And he tries to prepare these in ways that add no extra fat, such as poaching and steaming.

Czekelius learned about healthy cooking from a nutrition consultant in Boston, who taught him and his staff how to cut the fat in rich, classic dishes. Now he's using that knowledge to create low-fat, low-calorie, low-sodium dishes at this Cape Cod resort.

"I call my cooking 'honest cuisine,' " he says. "My feeling is that if you make nutrient claims on your menu, you should be scrupulous about following your guidelines in the kitchen. Use nutritious ingredients and measure them accurately."

As part of his continuing education, Czekelius is taking a nutrition course at the Culinary Institute of America. And he's so intent on imparting a respect for nutrition to the next generation of chefs that he's implemented an apprenticeship with an emphasis on healthy eating and cooking. "Nutrition is slowly but surely becoming part of the chef's repertoire," he says.

Cape Cod Scallops with Tomatoes

1¼ pounds sea scallops

3 tablespoons minced fresh parsley

2 tablespoons lemon juice

2 teaspoons chopped fresh basil or ½ teaspoon dried basil

1 teaspoon chopped fresh rosemary or ¼ teaspoon dried rosemary

1 teaspoon chopped fresh dill or ¼ teaspoon dillweed

1 clove garlic, minced

⅛ teaspoon black pepper

1 teaspoon olive oil

1 cup sliced onions

1 cup sliced sweet red and yellow peppers

1 cup sliced mushrooms

1½ cups peeled and diced tomatoes

1 cup fish stock or chicken broth

In a medium bowl, combine the scallops, parsley, lemon juice, basil, rosemary, dill, garlic, and black pepper. Marinate 2 hours in the refrigerator.

In a large nonstick frying pan over medium-high heat, heat the oil for 30 seconds. Add the onions and peppers and sauté for 5 minutes. Add the mushrooms and cook for 1 minute.

Add the tomatoes and stock. Bring to a simmer.

Drain and discard the lemon marinade from the scallops. Add the scallops to the frying pan. Simmer for 4 to 6 minutes. Using a slotted spoon, remove the scallops and vegetables to a platter. Increase the heat to high and boil the stock until reduced by half. Pour over the scallops.

Makes 4 servings (182 calories, 3 grams fat [15% of calories], 2 grams dietary fiber, 26 grams protein, 0.28 gram omega-3's, 47 milligrams cholesterol, 256 milligrams sodium per serving. Also a good source of vitamins B_{12} and C and phosphorus)

New England Fish Chowder

1 quart fish stock or chicken broth

2 large baking potatoes, quartered

2 leeks

1 cup sliced onions

1 tablespoon oil

3 cups water

6 small red potatoes, cubed

½ cup sliced celery

1 teaspoon dried tarragon

½ teaspoon dried thyme

   pinch of ground white pepper

1 pound cod or haddock fillets, cut into large chunks

12 clams, scrubbed

¼ pound lobster meat, chopped

1 cup low-fat milk or evaporated skim milk

2 tablespoons minced fresh parsley

2 tablespoons minced sweet red pepper

In a 2-quart saucepan combine the stock and baking potatoes. Bring to a boil over high heat, then reduce the heat to low and simmer for 20 minutes.

Cut the leeks in half lengthwise and wash thoroughly to remove any grit from between the layers. Thinly slice the leeks, using the white part.

Combine the leeks, onions, and oil in a small frying pan. Sauté over medium heat for 8 to 10 minutes, or until golden.

Transfer the leeks and onions to a blender. Add the cooked potatoes and stock. Process on high for 1 minute, or until smooth.

In a 3- or 4-quart saucepan, combine the water, red potatoes, celery, tarragon, thyme, and white pepper. Bring to a boil over high heat, then reduce the heat to low and simmer for 10 minutes. Add the cod or haddock, clams, and lobster. Simmer for 5 minutes. Stir in the milk and

puréed vegetables; simmer for 5 minutes. Serve garnished
with parsley and red pepper.

*Makes 6 servings (267 calories, 5 grams fat [17% of cal-
ories], 1 gram dietary fiber, 27 grams protein, 0.25 gram
omega-3's, 66 milligrams cholesterol, 159 milligrams sodium. Also a good source of vitamin C, iron, niacin, and
potassium)*

Chef August Mrozowski, Cafe L'Europe, Sarasota, Florida

Welcome to Cafe L'Europe, an elegant Gulf Coast restaurant that made a heartfelt commitment when chef August
Mrozowski unveiled his Light L'Europe menu. "We have
always cooked with a light touch, but this new menu sends
a clear message to the customer," he says. And the message
is that Cafe L'Europe is serious about nutrition.

Mrozowski enlisted a registered dietitian to help him
integrate good health with stylish food. The secret to the
lightness is substitution.

Regional specialties, such as red snapper, grouper, calico scallops, and crawfish, get new treatment. They're
steamed, poached, or grilled rather than fried. And they get
zip from Louisiana hot sauce or hot peppers rather than a
lot of salt. Healthy monounsaturated canola and olive oils
replace butter for light sautéing and form the base of vinai-
grettes and other dressings.

Each item on the menu follows American Heart Association guidelines. First the chef creates a recipe that
looks beautiful and tastes great. Then the dietitian makes
calorie, cholesterol, fat, and sodium calculations. If adjust-
ments are needed, the chef makes them. It works as a very
fluid arrangement between chef and nutritionist.

Mrozowski is so confident about the appeal and quality
of his menu that he prints the nutrient analysis for each
item on the Light L'Europe menu. And the emphasis on
nutrition is well appreciated by Cafe L'Europe's clientele.

Gulf Bouillabaisse

1 tablespoon olive oil

1 cup sliced carrots

1 cup sliced celery

1 cup sliced red onions

1 cup sliced fresh fennel

1 leek, sliced

1 pound tomatoes, peeled, seeded, and chopped

1 clove garlic, minced

$\frac{1}{4}$ teaspoon saffron threads

2 quarts stock

2 bay leaves

$\frac{1}{2}$ teaspoon fennel seeds

$\frac{1}{2}$ teaspoon dried oregano

$\frac{1}{8}$ teaspoon ground white pepper

1 2-inch strip orange rind

$1\frac{1}{4}$ pound grouper or red snapper, cut into 6 pieces

$\frac{3}{4}$ pound calico scallops or bay scallops

12 shrimp, peeled and deveined

12 whole crawfish

2 tablespoons minced fresh parsley

In a large pot over medium-high heat, heat the oil for 30 seconds. Add the carrots, celery, onions, fennel, and leeks and sauté for 5 minutes. Add the tomatoes, garlic, and saffron. Sauté for 5 minutes.

Add the stock, bay leaves, fennel seeds, oregano, white pepper, and orange rind. Bring to a boil, then reduce the heat, cover, and simmer for 30 minutes.

Add the grouper or snapper, scallops, shrimp, crawfish, and parsley. Cover and simmer for 5 to 7 minutes.

Makes 6 servings (280 calories, 7 grams fat [23% of calories], 2.7 grams dietary fiber, 36.7 grams protein, 0.39 gram omega-3's, 84 milligrams cholesterol, 346 milligrams sodium per serving. Also a good source of vitamins A, B_{12}, and C; magnesium; and potassium)

Steamed Red Snapper with Pepper Relish

1 sweet red pepper

1 yellow pepper

1 green pepper

2 tablespoons balsamic or sherry vinegar

1 tablespoon chopped fresh coriander

3 scallions, minced

2 teaspoons canola oil

½ teaspoon minced chili pepper or Louisiana hot pepper sauce

4 red snapper fillets (6 ounces each)

Broil the red, yellow, and green peppers for several minutes until the skins are dark and blistered. Turn them and continue broiling until all sides are blackened. Cool in a brown paper bag. Discard skins, cores, and seeds; dice flesh. Transfer to a medium bowl.

Add the vinegar, coriander, scallions, oil, and chili peppers or hot pepper sauce. Set aside.

Steam the fish over boiling water for 7 to 8 minutes. Serve with the pepper relish.

Makes 4 servings (202 calories, 5 grams fat [22% of calories], 0.6 gram dietary fiber, 35.2 grams protein, 0.5 gram omega-3's, 62 milligrams cholesterol, 110 milligrams sodium per serving. Also a good source of vitamin C, magnesium, and potassium)

Chef Caprial Pence, Fullers, Seattle, Washington

As head chef at the award-winning Fullers restaurant in the Seattle Sheraton, Caprial Pence has a talent for turning heart-healthy ingredients into exciting dishes. And Fullers restaurant has been a perfect showcase for her brand of culinary flair.

One of the healthiest types of fish is native to the Pacific Northwest: salmon. Varieties like coho and chinook are treasure troves of omega-3 fatty acids. Little wonder that they're regularly featured on Pence's celebrated menu. Other local flavor-filled ingredients she relies on include

Washington's sweet Walla Walla onions and wild mushrooms. They provide lots of oomph without extra fat, calories, or salt.

The restaurant's "Healthy Alternatives" menu is the product of Caprial's collaboration with a dietitian. Together they fashioned heart-healthy culinary delights that are a big success with patrons. Although a nutrient analysis is not printed on the menu, it's readily available from the kitchen.

Pence's patrons appreciate the effort. Recently, for instance, one asked for "sautéed" shrimp prepared without fat. Caprial improvised, puréeing rhubarb with ginger, shallots, and garlic, then briefly heating it as a sauce for the shrimp. The woman was so delighted that she sent friends over the following night for the same dish.

A few years ago Pence had to make the choice between a culinary career and one in medicine. With the work she's doing at Fullers, she's blended the best of both professions.

Grilled Salmon with Cucumber Relish

½ cup diced red onions

½ cup rice wine vinegar

2 shallots, minced

2 cloves garlic, minced

1 teaspoon peeled minced gingerroot

1 teaspoon grated orange rind

¼ teaspoon low-sodium soy sauce

2 cucumbers, quartered lengthwise and thinly sliced

⅛ teaspoon ground white pepper

4 salmon fillets (6 ounces each)

2 teaspoons olive oil

2 cups hot cooked rice

In a large nonstick frying pan over medium-high heat, combine the onions, vinegar, shallots, garlic, ginger, orange rind, and soy sauce. Bring the mixture to a boil, stir, and cook for 30 seconds. Remove from the heat.

Add the cucumbers and pepper. Set aside to cool.

Add the cucumbers and pepper. Set aside to cool.

Rub the salmon with the oil and grill or broil for 4 to 5 minutes per side. Serve on a bed of rice. Spoon the cucumber relish over the fish.

Makes 4 servings (407 calories, 13.3 grams fat [29% of calories], 3 grams dietary fiber, 37 grams protein, 2.9 grams omega-3's, 94 milligrams cholesterol, 95 milligrams sodium per serving. Also a good source of vitamins B_6 and B_{12}, niacin, riboflavin, thiamine, and potassium)

Halibut with Roasted Garlic and Wild Mushrooms

1 whole garlic bulb, unpeeled

1 tablespoon sherry vinegar

1 tablespoon water

2 shallots, minced

1 tablespoon olive oil

½ cup sliced shiitake or other available mushrooms

3 Italian tomatoes, diced

⅛ teaspoon black pepper

¾ cup stock or white wine

  juice of 1 lemon

2 cloves garlic, crushed

¼ teaspoon dried thyme

4 halibut steaks (6 ounces each)

Roast the garlic bulb at 400°F for 10 to 15 minutes. Break the bulb into cloves. Peel three of the cloves, chop, and place in a medium bowl. (Reserve the remainder for another use.)

Add the vinegar, water, and shallots. Whisk in the oil. Add the mushrooms, tomatoes, and pepper. Set aside.

In a large pot, combine the stock or wine, lemon juice, crushed garlic, and thyme. Bring to a boil.

Place the halibut on a steamer rack in the pan. Cover and steam for 7 to 10 minutes. Remove from the pan. (Reserve the steaming liquid for another use.)

Divide vegetables among four dinner plates. Top with halibut steaks.

Makes 4 servings (209 calories, 6.8 grams fat [30% of calories], 0.4 gram dietary fiber, 31 grams protein, 45 milligrams cholesterol, 0.57 gram omega-3's, 99 milligrams sodium per serving. Also a good source of vitamins B_6 and B_{12} and niacin)

How to Buy and Make the Best

Simplify. That's the message from the guest chefs. Learn a few basic techniques, they say, and you'll never be intimidated by fish cookery again. Their rules: Buy the best. Never overcook it. Here's how.

Buying • When buying whole fish, look for ruby red gills, firm flesh, clear eyes, and moist scales; fillets should have a fresh odor, never "fishy." Buy fish last, then rush it home and refrigerate or cook it promptly. If you must store fish for a day, wash with cold water, wrap in plastic, and put on ice in the fridge.

Steaming • For cod, flounder, grouper, haddock, halibut, mahimahi, pollock, red snapper, rockfish, salmon, scrod, sea bass, sole, and walleye:

1. Bring 1 cup liquid to a boil in wok or large pot with tight lid.
2. Place fish on steaming rack coated with nonstick spray. Add to pot.
3. Cover with lid and steam 10 minutes. Do not remove lid until time is up.

Some suggested steaming liquids: lemongrass tea; lemon verbena tea; water with 1 tablespoon Dijon mustard, 1 tablespoon lemon juice, and 1 teaspoon thyme.

Poaching • For catfish, cod, flounder, haddock, halibut, mahimahi, monkfish, orange roughy, pollock, pout, red snapper, salmon, scrod, sole, trout (whole), and walleye:

1. Bring 6 cups water or bouillon and herbs or spices to boil over medium-high heat; boil 5 minutes.
2. Add fish and additional water to cover. Reduce heat to a simmer. Cook 10 minutes.

A suggested poaching liquid: 6 cups water, 3 tablespoons wine vinegar, 12 peppercorns, 5 parsley sprigs, 3 bay leaves. If desired, boil down the liquid, strain, and use as a brothy sauce.

Baking • For bluefish, catfish, cod, flounder, grouper, haddock, halibut, mackerel, mahimahi, orange roughy, pollock, red snapper, rockfish, salmon, scrod, sea trout, sole, and trout (whole):

1. Brush fish with juice. Sprinkle with bread crumbs.
2. Place on baking sheet. Bake at 400°F for 6 minutes.
3. Baste with more juice. Bake 6 minutes.

A suggested juice: 2 tablespoons each of orange, lemon, and lime juice.

Grilling • For catfish, grouper, halibut, marlin, monkfish, red snapper, rockfish, sablefish, salmon, shark, swordfish, tilefish, tuna:

1. Place marinated fish on very hot grill; cover with lid.
2. Cook 3 to 4 minutes. Use spatula to reposition fish at 45-degree angle to original (do not flip fish).
3. Cover and cook 3 to 4 minutes.

A suggested marinade: 2 tablespoons lime juice, 1 tablespoon canola oil; cover and refrigerate 30 minutes.

And here are a few serving suggestions.

• Top a simply prepared fish with a flavorful vinaigrette: Mix chopped tomato, minced roasted garlic, olive oil, and sherry vinegar.
• Or, for a main-course salad, add grilled fish to a tossed salad. Dress with vinaigrette of raspberry vinegar, canola oil, and chicken stock.
• Accompany fish with vegetable or fruit relish: Chop sweet peppers, tomatoes, or mangoes. Toss with hot vinegar, honey, and scallions. Let stand 1 hour before using.
• Splash on flavored vinegars, such as raspberry, cabernet wine, or rice wine, after the fish is cooked.

Natural
Tranquilizers

Stop Panic Attacks
in Their Tracks

Fast, shallow breathing; sudden, intense feelings of fearfulness with no obvious cause—a panic attack. Most physicians agree that people in the midst of a panic attack hyperventilate in response to the intense anxiety they feel.

But new evidence suggests that, in some people, hyperventilation may actually occur *before* the panic attack, triggering the fears that accompany such an episode. In fact, David H. Barlow, Ph.D., director of the Center for Stress and Anxiety Disorders at the State University of New York at Albany, believes that *hyperventilation is the primary problem in about half of panic-attack victims.*

For these people, the symptoms most often caused by hyperventilation—light-headedness, dizziness, breathlessness—trigger feelings of anxiety. This anxiety fuels their already out-of-control breathing, which continues to increase in intensity until full-fledged panic takes hold.

What they're suffering from is chronic hyperventilation syndrome (CHS), a new diagnosis describing those for whom hyperventilation has become an unrecognized but devastating habit.

"Panic attacks" are just one possible symptom of CHS. Experts estimate that as many as one in ten people who walk into a doctor's office are suffering from CHS. Their symptoms range from feelings of panic to light-headedness; tingling and coldness in the fingers, face, and feet;

excessive yawning; belching; fatigue—and even chest pains that give the appearance of a heart attack.

CHS sufferers come in fearing they have a psychological problem or heart disease. They go through a lengthy battery of tests with psychologists, cardiologists, neurologists—even allergists. Some never find out what's wrong with them. Others are branded hypochondriacs.

"The *worst* thing that can happen is for the doctor to say, 'It's all in your head,' " says John H. Renner, M.D., a consumer health expert at Trinity Lutheran Hospital in Kansas City. Dr. Renner has treated many of his own patients for CHS and, he assures us, "Symptoms of chronic hyperventilation are *very* real."

How the Bad Breathing Habit Gets Started

Researchers at King's College School of Medicine and Dentistry in London (writing in the *British Journal of Hospital Medicine*) say that habitual bad breathing may result from conditions as varied as mild asthma, chronic bronchitis, protracted pain, anxiety, and depression.

Other experts add that a lengthy period of high stress, like drawn-out divorce proceedings or financial problems, can cause a person to start the hyperventilation habit, which often lingers long after those original problems are gone.

In fact, almost anything can get a bad breathing habit started. Dr. Renner cites the case of a man who began breathing lightly while his chest was taped to heal broken ribs. The breathing style that eased his pain remained behind and led to CHS after the tape was removed.

Those prone to CHS may hyperventilate when they are tired or under stress, during or after exercise, while falling asleep or waking up, or even periodically throughout the day. This kind of a hyperventilation habit causes a person to give off more carbon dioxide when they exhale than they should. This in turns causes carbon dioxide levels in the blood to drop, because you're exhaling stuff that should stay in your blood to give it a good mix of the gases that it naturally contains.

And people with low blood levels of carbon dioxide are

always on the threshold of experiencing symptoms, says Dr. Renner. Any increase in breathing—yawning, exercising, even laughter—can drop those levels down into the danger zone and release a real Pandora's box of symptoms—including panic attack.

Do *You* Hyperventilate?

It's not easy to tell if you're hyperventilating. Have you ever actually *tried* to pay attention to your breathing? It's almost a contradiction in terms! You can't suddenly start thinking about something that you're supposed to do unconsciously without screwing it up.

"As soon as you focus on any automatic body function, like breathing, it's going to speed up," explains Dr. Barlow. So trying to "time" your normal breathing isn't the answer.

Shallow breathing, on the other hand, *is* detectable. If your breathing is too shallow, you'll notice that your stomach doesn't move when you inhale; only your chest heaves.

Proper breathing—that allows your lungs to fill all the way up with air—forces your stomach to move as well.

Don't Hold Your Breath; Take This Test!

Lie down and place one hand on your chest and one on your stomach, just above your navel. If the hand on your stomach doesn't move at all while you inhale, you are breathing from your chest.

Of course, shallow breathing alone won't bring on chronic hyperventilation symptoms. You also have to breathe rapidly.

If you're a rapid breather, you may often feel like you're not getting enough air. You yawn or sigh a lot. When frightened, you hold your breath, then breathe out hard afterward.

The definitive CHS self-test is described by Dr. Barlow in his book, *Mastery of Your Anxiety and Panic*. All that's involved is deliberate overbreathing—inhaling and exhaling quickly in rapid succession.

If such rapid breathing causes you to experience previously unexplained symptoms like chest pain, panicky feelings, dizziness, light-headedness, tingling in the fingers, and chronic belching or bloating, then there's a good chance that your "mystery" symptoms have been CHS induced.

For safety's sake, however, don't do this alone. Arrange to try it first in your doctor's office so you can be monitored during the test. People with heart disease or serious lung ailments like emphysema could suffer an adverse reaction to such intense breathing, and you don't want to hurt yourself for the sake of a diagnosis.

Besides, if your doctor actually *sees* it happen, it'll help him or her to understand the true nature of your problem and better enable him or her to work with you on the solution; which is . . .

Learning How to Breathe Better

The best way to teach yourself to breathe properly is to spend several weeks performing exercises similar to the deep breathing taught in yoga classes. Dr. Barlow uses such a system to help people who are suffering from anxiety attacks and feels that it helps hyperventilators as well.

Phase One—Belly Breathing • During the first phase, you learn how to breathe from your stomach. Lie face down on the floor with your head sideways, resting on your cheek. Learn to push your stomach against the floor each time you inhale.

After you've done that for a while, turn over and place a book on your stomach. Try to raise the book with each inhalation.

If you habitually breathe from your chest, breathing from your stomach may make you feel a little out of control at first. Just relax, remind yourself that you're in no danger and the feeling will pass. Once you're comfortable with the basics of belly breathing, begin regular practice sessions.

Sit in a quiet, comfortable place and give yourself a few seconds to relax. Then, start counting with your inhalations. Think "one" to yourself as you breathe in, then "relax" as you breathe out; "two" in, "relax" out. Keep going until you reach ten, then return to one.

Repeat this counting sequence for 10 minutes, twice a day, every day for one week. During this first phase of the program, don't try to change the speed or depth of your breathing. (You should *always* breathe through your nose. It's the proper way to do things, *and* it can be a big help if you feel the urge to speed up your breathing.)

If you feel like you are not getting enough air, try pushing your stomach out just a little before you inhale.

Phase Two—Slowing Down • Start slowing your breathing by matching it to your counting. Say the number to yourself and *then* inhale. Think "relax" and then exhale. Slow the counting rate a little each day until you are taking ten breaths a minute (inhaling for 3 seconds, then exhaling for 3 seconds).

You'll know you've reached the proper breathing rate when you can say "one thousand one, one thousand two, one thousand three" to yourself during one inhalation or exhalation. Check yourself occasionally with one hand on your chest and one on your stomach to make sure you're still breathing correctly.

Practice for 10 minutes twice a day for one week.

Now that you've practiced for a total of two weeks in calm, quiet surroundings, you're ready for . . .

Phase Three—Going Public • Now it's time to use your breathing technique throughout the day—at work, while you're shopping and—especially—in stressful situations.

Each time, count from one to ten and back down to one again. Don't get discouraged if your control isn't as good now that you're using it in real-life situations.

Trust that you have the skill, and that you will get better at using it with practice. Continue the twice-a-day practice sessions as well. Regular practice helps train your lungs to breathe normally throughout the day.

But be *sure* you use the counting technique whenever you're under stress. That, say the experts, is when it *really* counts.

Calm Down Quickly, Easily, Naturally

The boss glared at you this morning. The automatic teller machine insisted you had no account and wouldn't return your bank card. Your son says you got an "urgent" message from someone named either "Ira" or "the IRS."

Let's face it, you can't avoid stressful situations. Your best defense is to diffuse the tension as quickly as possible—not with drugs or a stiff drink, but preferably with a natural "tranquilizer"—something that will settle your nerves but won't dampen your verve or clobber you with an assortment of unwanted side effects.

Some of the six techniques discussed here have been tested against Valium, one of the most common tranquilizing drugs, and proven effective. Remember: These are fast and natural tension relievers to counter everyday stress. If your anxiety persists or becomes extreme, consult your doctor.

Blow Up at Stress

If you don't want to crack under stress, try cracking up: A hearty laugh is universally considered one of the best ways to puncture stress. But it's often difficult to force a laugh in a tense moment. But experts have come up with a technique that does the trick—any time, any place. Allen Elkin, Ph.D., program director of Stresscare Systems, Inc., a Long Island company that conducts stress management seminars, calls it the "blow-up method." It's a tension diffuser that involves blowing a situation out of proportion—to the point of ludicrousness. It can prompt a laugh and diffuse a volatile situation.

Here's how it works. Let's say you're in a traffic jam. Bumper-to-bumper. Instead of fuming in silence, talk out the most horrible scenario you can imagine. "I'll be stuck here for hours. These cars will never move. They'll have to close the freeway and airlift us out of here. Of course, they'll probably have one helicopter to airlift thousands of cars. By the time they get to me, my children will have grown up, married, and had children of their own. No one will even remember who I am.''

''By exaggerating the situation to the point of absurdity you begin to smile at yourself. This helps you put a situation into perspective,'' says Dr. Elkin. And perspective is a natural calmer because stress is usually caused not by a situation, but by how we perceive a situation.

Mellow Out with Music

Maybe music really can soothe the savage breast. The research in this area is very sketchy, but several scientists theorize that playing calming music in operating rooms may reduce the amount of anesthesia patients need, and that music can help tranquilize people undergoing dental work.

Most experts say relaxation music should be slow, quiet, and nonvocal, since lyrics may also influence mood negatively. But don't despair if you're bored by Bach. Cheryl D. Maranto, Ph.D., president of the National Association for Music Therapy, says the two most important characteristics of tranquilizing music may be ''familiarity and preference.'' Experiment to see what works best for you. Sit quietly with your eyes closed and breathe slowly (inhale for a count of four, exhale for a count of four) while listening to the music. Imagine the notes flowing over you like a waterfall, rinsing away tension and leaving you feeling refreshed.

Walk Away from Tension

More than a decade ago, a 15-minute walk was found to have a greater calming effect than the tranquilizer meprobamate. Researchers are now beginning to learn just how far a short walk can distance you from your anxiety.

Robert Thayer, Ph.D., professor of psychology at California State University, Long Beach, has done several studies of the effects of a brisk, 10-minute walk. Dr. Thayer reports that subjects felt less tense and more energetic after walking (as measured by questionnaires).

In one study, 18 subjects were each given a candy bar to eat, then 30, 60, and 120 minutes afterward were asked to describe how they felt. Next, the subjects took a brisk walk and again, after 30, 60, and 120 minutes, were asked to describe how tense or relaxed they felt. After walking, people noticed more energy and less tension than after eating the candy bar. And the effect lasted for 2 hours.

Dr. Thayer found that students who walked on a treadmill in a bare room reported roughly the same tension reduction as those who walked around a scenic campus. He suspects that chemicals released in the brain during a walk may be responsible.

Another study suggests that it's how you walk, not where, that makes a difference. Sara Snodgrass, Ph.D., professor of psychology at Skidmore College in Saratoga Springs, New York, had a total of 79 students walk for 3 minutes in three different manners: using their normal gait; taking long strides, swinging their arms, and looking forward; and shuffling along with their eyes downward. Psychological tests measured the students' own sense of fatigue and depression (psychological factors that can be associated with stress). Results revealed that the shufflers' moods were worse than those who walked in their regular stride. One possible reason: "When you swing your arms there's a kind of mechanical action that soothes the muscles in the shoulders, neck, and back, which are often tense when we are anxious," says Dr. Thayer, author of *The Biopsychology of Mood and Arousal.*

To walk off tension, then, Dr. Thayer offers these tips: Clear your mind, pretend your head is held up by a helium-filled balloon, breathe naturally, and let your arms swing freely at your sides.

Talk It Out

Nervous about giving a speech? Talk about it. Going through a divorce? Share your anxiety. Afraid you're going to lose your job? Tell someone. By voicing your fear, you clarify it for yourself and gain perspective. Sometimes, too, a listener (especially one who's experienced the same problem) can dispel the sense of isolation that often compounds the emotional stress.

"Often what causes stress and tension are the things we keep inside," says Jerilyn Ross, president of the Phobia Society of America and associate director of the Roundhouse Square Psychiatric Center in Alexandria, Virginia. "Identify someone in your life who you can talk to when you're starting to feel anxious."

Are there times you should keep your lips zipped? Of course. Here are some guidelines for positive confession from Ross and other experts: Confide only in someone who has your best interests at heart. Talk to someone who really listens; if you sense the listener is bored or distracted, you're probably right. And watch sudden impulses to talk: If you decide to confide a problem, wait an hour and see if it still feels right. If so, go ahead. What if you feel too uncomfortable to talk about your problem? Write down your feelings in a letter and then throw the letter away. Or speak your mind into a tape recorder, then erase the tape. To relieve 3:00 A.M. anxiety, get out of bed, write down the problem, put the paper in an envelope, and say you will deal with it tomorrow morning at 9:30. Dr. Elkin of Stresscare says by making an appointment with yourself for a "worry time" you remove a major part of the problem: deciding to deal with it.

Soak Away Anxiety

In days past, hot baths were commonly used to tranquilize institutionalized mental patients. Today, few would be advised to hop into hot water. The most relaxing baths are warm—about 100° to 102°F, says Carole B. Lewis, Ph.D., adjunct associate professor at the University of Pittsburgh and associate professor of medicine at George Washington University, in Washington, D.C. Hot water shocks the system, causing muscles to constrict. Warm water calms you by increasing circulation and relaxing muscles, she says. (In one study, researchers theorize that heating the body may even cause biochemical changes that induce deeper sleep.) And to enhance the tranquilizing effect of a warm bath combine it with a form of progressive relaxation.

"First let your hand gently float on the water," says Dr. Lewis. "To do this, your hand must be completely relaxed." Then imagine that feeling of relaxation in your hand moving up to your elbow, along your arm and to your head. Let it work its luxurious, soothing power into the places in your body where you hold tension. Then go down to your feet and start again, slowly moving up your body.

One caution: If you are taking vasoconstricting blood pressure medicine, check with your doctor before taking the bathtub plunge.

Shift Respiration into Auto-Relax

When anxiety strikes, the heart races and breathing becomes shallow and rapid. But, by reversing the symptoms of stress—by breathing slowly and deeply—you can calm yourself almost instantly.

Deep breathing causes your body to release endorphins, which are tranquilizing hormones. Best of all, it takes just 30 seconds to bring about the calming effect.

The technique is simple. Slowly breathe in through your nose, comfortably expanding your abdomen first and then your rib cage. (Imagine you're inflating a beach ball in your stomach through your belly button, says Dr. Elkin.) Then release the breath through your nose (more slowly than you let it in) and silently say, "Relax" or "Let go."

Once you've mastered this technique, you may be able to train your respiratory system to relax on cue, says Jeffrey A. Migdow, M.D., instructor at Kripalu Center for Yoga and Health in Lenox, Massachusetts, and coauthor of *Take a Deep Breath*. Set cues for yourself to breathe deeply for a minute or two throughout the day—whenever your office door closes or the phone rings, for example. Then, when you get home, practice the deep-breathing technique for 10 minutes.

After a few months, perhaps even weeks, you'll automatically begin breathing slowly and deeply during tense moments.

The Mood/Music Connection

By Robert Ornstein, Ph.D., and David Sobel, M.D.

You are sitting in a darkened room. At moments you feel intense, spine-tingling thrills, which seem to begin at your neck and radiate over your head and all the way down to your toes. You actually shiver with pleasure and get goose bumps; you may even weep. What could possibly be the source of such delicious sensations? Fabulous sex? A well-wrought movie? A glorious painting? The birth of a great idea?

Had you participated in this study at Stanford University, you would have been responding to music.

Music can be an intense as well as a healthy pleasure. Indeed, one survey showed that some of us find music more thrilling than anything else—including sex (which tied with nostalgic moments for sixth place on the all-time thrill scale).

And at least part of the thrill of music may come from the release of endorphins, powerful opiate-like chemicals produced in the brain that relieve pain and induce euphoria. When a drug is administered that blocks these pleasure-releasing chemicals, some of the thrills of listening to music are significantly blunted.

You don't have to be musically inclined to be influenced by music. By choice or by chance, music is a part of your life—beginning, in a way, before you were born, with the rhythm of your mother's beating heart. Her voice is the beginning of a lullaby. Perhaps Muzak is an ersatz lullaby for adults—soothing us unaware in elevators, at the dentist, in banks—persuading us to joyfully hand over our credit cards in shopping centers and department stores.

Find Your Mood Movers

Almost all of us have a musical preference, playing "radio roulette," tapping feet in time to music, singing along with a favorite tune at the top of our lungs. We don't have to splurge for a subscription to the symphony, retreat under headphones, or go to church to tune in to how music affects us. Be it Bach, jazz, rock, gospel, or pop, music is a mood mover. The right music at the right time brings us joy and serenity and soothes frazzled nerves. It lifts us up when we're down and calms us when we're too excited. It can move us to tears, or get us in the mood to eat, study, work, or make love.

We seem to have a built-in response to certain tones: People uniformly describe high-pitched music as happy and playful, low-pitched music as sad and serious. On the other hand, tempo may be the most important factor for our heart and our head.

Our heart normally beats between 70 and 80 times per minute. Most western music is set (coincidentally?) to this tempo. Some studies have shown that heart rate synchronizes with music, speeding up or slowing down accordingly. Music also alters the brain's electrical rhythms.

Music influences respiratory rate, blood pressure, stomach contractions, and the level of stress hormones in the blood. Although people react differently, slow, quiet, nonvocal music generally lowers bodily reactions to stress, while the faster variety heightens alertness and arousal. Perhaps some of music's allure stems simply from its ability to distract us from less pleasant thoughts and feelings, albeit temporarily.

Distraction may partly explain why exercise feels better to music—because it helps us gain with less pain. One study showed that moving to an even rhythm made muscles flex and extend more smoothly. And music may get you in tune with your body, increasing endurance, regulating breathing, and getting you in the mood to exercise. With upbeat rock music, exercisers tend to feel as if they haven't worked as hard.

Brahms Valium

If the thought of surgery, hospitalization, or the dentist's drill sends chills up and down your spine, you may be able to transcend them with sound.

When music is played for patients before, during, or after surgery, it has been found to reduce anxiety, lessen pain, reduce need for preoperative and postoperative medication, and speed recovery. In one study, when soothing music was piped into an operating room throughout surgery, the amount of sedative required by patients was cut in half.

The patients were generally enthusiastic about the experience, remarking "It was very enjoyable indeed," "I heard Pachelbel's 'Canon' when I awoke, and it was a nice, underlying thing." Not exactly a typical postoperative reaction. In another study, the investigator estimated that music had an effect comparable to that of an intravenous dose of 2.5 milligrams of Valium.

"Musical Valium" has worked for male and female, young and old, and in patients undergoing a wide variety of surgical procedures, from tubal ligation to spinal fusion. Two studies conducted on surgical patients in Japan indicate that listening to music before and during surgery reduces the level of stress hormones in the blood. Since surrounding noises and voices in the operating room are a common source of anxiety for patients—even those who receive general anesthesia may be able to hear them—part of the beneficial effect may be due to the music blocking out these distressing sounds.

Now you know why you're subjected to "dentist music." When played during a variety of dental treatments, including drilling and tooth extraction, an earful of music enhances the effect of the anesthetic.

Music can even make childbirth a more pleasant experience. When combined with Lamaze exercises, music has been shown to reduce the pain and duration of labor by as much as 2 hours, while enhancing the euphoria of birth.

So the next time you or someone you know is scheduled for a dental or medical procedure, consider bringing or requesting music.

Take Two Arias and Call Me in the Morning

Music as medical therapy began in ancient times. The oldest known medical document is a papyrus that refers to incantations used to heal the sick. To the ancient Greeks, Apollo was the god of music. Early physicians used music to regulate heartbeat, and music and singing were traditionally used to cure many ailments, including melancholia. Healing with sound, rhythm, and chanting is widely accepted in many cultures throughout the world.

Our culture's version of music therapy helps people cope with the emotional and physical effects of many types of illness. Helen Bonny, Ph.D., music therapist and former director of music therapy at the Catholic University of America in Washington, D.C., has used music to facilitate psychotherapy, but when she developed heart disease, she turned to music to help heal herself.

She knew firsthand how important music could be to vulnerable hospital patients trapped in a cold, sterile, often boring environment. She began her pilot project by piping quiet music into the intensive coronary care units of two hospitals. The music reduced heart rates, lowered blood pressure, increased pain tolerance, and lessened anxiety and depression.

Music therapy is a useful adjunct in the treatment of many illnesses, including cancer, respiratory problems, stroke, arthritis, and diabetes. It's used to ease the administration and counteract the side effects of such potentially unpleasant treatments as chemotherapy, radiation, and kidney dialysis. It works to ease the pain, calm the anxiety, and lift the spirits of the terminally or chronically ill.

Medicine for the Emotions

Music is used extensively for treatment of diseases like headaches, digestive problems, and depression, which have a strong emotional component. It has also been successful in breaking through to autistic children.

Music is also used to reduce depression, anxiety, and isolation in burn victims, organ transplant patients, and people with contagious diseases, who spend long periods of time in otherwise sterile environments. A particularly bittersweet application is reaching comatose or brain-damaged patients.

One 13-year-old auto-accident victim appeared comatose and wasn't responding to anyone or anything. He gradually responded to a variety of music. His therapy began with the simple act of turning his head toward the music. Eventually, he sang and played musical instruments. Before he was discharged from the hospital $4\frac{1}{2}$ months after the accident, he said to his music therapist, "Music makes me happy."

Music may also be nourishing for premature infants. When Brahms's "Lullaby" was prescribed for these babies, the results were striking. The infants gained weight faster and were able to leave the hospital an average of one week sooner than the babies who didn't hear the music, at a savings of $4,800 per infant.

Musical Immunity

If music can make such a difference in the outcome of medical procedures, illness, and treatment, what are its benefits in supporting good health and preventing illness in people who are basically healthy to begin with?

An answer may lie in the effect of music on immune function. High levels of stress hormones appear to suppress our immune system, but music may help control these hormones.

Music therapist and researcher Mark Rider studied night- and rotating-shift hospital nurses who suffered health problems due to the stress produced from working at odd hours. The nurses listened to a 20-minute tape of relaxation exercises, guided imagery, and mellow music.

During the days of musical relaxation, the nurses' stress-hormone levels rose less steeply and their biological rhythms were more in sync. Interestingly, two of the subjects remarked that although at one point during the study they felt as though they were getting sick, they felt better after playing the music/relaxation tape.

We can make the effort to put more music in our lives, in either a structured or informal way.

Experiment with music and mood. Play a new or familiar recording and do nothing but listen, perhaps lying down in a darkened room.

Does it relax you? Stimulate you? Does it evoke a certain mood, feeling, memory, or image? Try measuring your pulse before, during, and after listening.

You might want to try some music that takes advantage of your mood—start with tense music to match your mood, and then use a piece that gradually makes the transition to more soothing sounds. This has been effective in reducing chronic pain.

If you are in pain or a particularly anxious mood, listening to soft, quiet music may at first clash with your feelings. If the music first matches your mood and resonates with your physiological state, however, it can lead you to a more relaxed state as you get in sync with it. A few soothing suggestions: Bach's "Air on the G String," Pachelbel's "Canon in D," Haydn's "Cello Concerto in C," and Debussy's "Claire de Lune." But personal reactions and preferences differ, so experiment.

Over 2,500 years ago, the Greek philosopher Pythagoras may have been on to something. He advocated daily singing and playing of an instrument as a cathartic to cleanse the emotions of worry, sorrow, fear, and anger.

Learning to play a musical instrument can increase the pleasure you get from music and give you a sense of mastery and pride in your accomplishment. And while a sonata a day may not keep the doctor away, it will probably feel good regardless. Enjoying music is an easy way to reclaim some of the sensuality lost in our lives.

Maximum Immunity

What a Little Walking Can Do

The toughest, meanest disease fighter on earth doesn't wear a white lab coat or lurk in a green pill or percolate in a test tube. It's in you. It's your immune system. Minute by minute, year by year, it slaughters more germs and deters more illness than you can imagine. So a lot of people want to know: What can you do to dial it up to full power, to ensure that it functions at the maximum?

One answer is good nutrition. Another may be stress reduction. But now science is exploring a new possibility, an exciting hypothesis that has researchers scrambling for clues: exercise.

Can You Walk Away from Colds?

Here's an example of the kind of fascinating research that's emerging. In a small-scale study from Loma Linda University, in California, researchers examined the possible effects of walking on the immune function and infectious illness rate of 50 moderately obese women who were not in an exercise program. The women were divided into two groups. One remained sedentary. The other group walked 45 minutes a day, five days a week, for 15 weeks during the winter and spring. All the women were asked to report any colds and flu, and immunity factors in the blood were checked along the way. (Our immune response is led by cells and proteins in our bloodstream that seek and destroy invading bacteria, viruses, parasites, or fungi.)

192

During the 15-week period, the walking women were sick for an average of five days—but the sedentary group was sick for twice as long. Another interesting finding: The activity of natural killer (NK) cells and other immune cells in the bloodstream increased in the walking group from the beginning of the study. (NK cells kill tumor cells and virus-infected cells.)

What's going on here?

It's actually too early to tell—this study and other preliminary research on the exercise/immunity connection is just barely scratching the surface. But one theory about how something as simple as walking could be affecting the immune system centers around hormones and hormonelike substances in the body called neurohormones (or neurotransmitters). They're produced both by the brain and the nervous and endocrine systems. These substances are not only responsible for communications in the brain and the nervous system, but also, scientists have discovered, appear to have the ability to turn on or turn off cells in the immune system. And moderate exercise, like walking, causes changes in certain neurotransmitters and hormones.

If you're a regular exerciser, you've probably experienced the pleasurable feelings of "runner's high" or "walker's high." These good feelings are believed to be caused by neurotransmitters called endorphins. There is some evidence that endorphins also aid the activity of certain immune cells.

Besides affecting neurotransmitters, exercise also temporarily increases levels of several other immune-stimulating substances, including interleukin-1. Interleukin-1 is a protein that stimulates the activity of T-cells (white blood cells, or lymphocytes, that identify threats and call other immune cells to arms) and B-cells (which produce proteins called antibodies that kill invaders). Interleukin-1 also raises body temperature. In animals, fever has been shown to enhance recovery from infections. (Some researchers hypothesize that the rise in temperature during exercise may help to provide an environment hostile to some viruses and bacteria.)

A change in (actually a decrease in the rise of) neuro-transmitters and hormones or an increase in other immune-stimulating substances could explain why the walking women in the Loma Linda study enjoyed an apparent boost in immunity from their moderate exercise. "If you exercise within your tolerance and training capacity, then it appears that may actually temporarily enhance certain aspects of immunity. The animal studies and a few human studies suggest that may be the situation," concludes Thomas Tomasi, M.D., Ph.D., an immunologist who heads the Roswell Park Cancer Institute in Buffalo, New York.

A major goal of this research is to figure out if the short-term rise in defending substances in the bloodstream translates into less illness for people in the long run. For some experts, this possibility is simply an additional plus for walking and other regular moderate exercise, which already have plenty of proven healthful effects going for them.

So far, though, the possibility is just that. No one knows for sure. In part this is because many studies don't take into account that the people who exercise may also acquire other lifestyle changes that may promote health.

Too Much of a Good Thing?

Whatever the discoveries made in the exercise/immunity connection, scientists are pretty sure about this: Moderate exercise like walking is better for immunity than the strenuous workouts of competition.

Current research indicates that too much exercise impairs immunity. "We think that excessive exercise acts like other forms of stress—and stress has been reported by many scientists to be detrimental to immunity," says Dr. Tomasi.

Athletic coaches have long believed that their athletes are particularly susceptible to illness immediately after a competition. Some even put their athletes into isolation for the hours immediately after an event. Dr. Tomasi found evidence for this belief in his studies of nationally ranked Nordic skiers and of competitive bicyclists asked to cycle to exhaustion in a laboratory. After the athletes' ordeals, Dr. Tomasi's researchers measured levels of antibodies in the saliva and NK cells in the bloodstream. They found a dramatic, although temporary, drop. "What we found was that when you are in a severe competition such as the national ski races, or when you push people in the laboratory 'to the wall'—where there's maximum exertion over a prolonged period—that harms certain aspects of the immune response," says Dr. Tomasi.

The Loma Linda researchers have come to similar conclusions. Their study of runners in the 1987 Los Angeles Marathon strongly suggests that "overdoing" exercise can cause higher rates of infectious illness. The scientists sent surveys to 4,900 runners who had registered for the race, asking them about illnesses. There were 2,300 respondents. Thirteen percent of the respondents who applied for the race and actually participated in the event reported becoming sick with colds, flu, or upper respiratory infections soon afterward. But of those runners who applied for the race and then decided not to run, only 2 percent later became sick. The runners who trained for 60-plus miles a week were more than twice as likely to become sick as those who trained for less than 20 miles a week.

The scientists followed up the survey with a laboratory marathon. Ten highly fit marathoners ran treadmill marathons. It was discovered that NK cell activity was depressed for up to 6 hours after their noncompetitive 26-mile runs.

Why might heavy exercise suppress immunity? Exercise to the point of exhaustion produces large amounts of hormones and neurotransmitters like cortisol and epinephrine. These substances, unlike those that aid immunity, are part of the classic stress response, says Loma Linda's Lee Berk, D.H.Sc. They're the reason we feel shaky, our blood pressure soars, and our heart pounds under stress, whether it's an automobile collision or an exhausting run.

The stress hormones and neurotransmitters impair the activity of certain immune cells, such as NK cells. David Neiman, D.H.Sc., chairman of the health science department at Loma Linda, who led the research team, notes that cortisol levels in the laboratory marathon runners were elevated by more than 50 percent for 1 to 1½ hours after the run. It wasn't until 2 to 3 hours after the laboratory marathons that cortisol levels fell, and NK cell levels were still depressed 6 hours after the marathon. (All runners' NK levels, however, were back to normal within 24 hours.) This research offers support to athletes' belief that there's a "window of opportunity" for illness to strike, when their training is the heaviest and after a competition.

Exercise and Cancer

A study of fitness and life span from the Institute for Aerobic Research in Dallas, Texas, made banner headlines. That study, published in the *Journal of the American Medical Association,* measured physical fitness of some 10,000 men and 3,000 women. The subjects were followed for eight years, and their death rates and causes tracked.

The researchers found dramatically lower mortality rates among the fitter participants. A key finding of the study was that even relatively low levels of fitness correlated with significantly increased longevity. Such levels of fitness are equivalent to what someone would reach if he or she took a brisk walk for at least a half hour a day every day.

But there was an even more remarkable finding. Not only were the fitter men and women less likely to die of cardiovascular disease—which is not surprising, given exercise's known benefits for strengthening the heart—but they were also less likely to die of cancer.

Cancer? Why would exercise and fitness level correlate with decreased risk of cancer? "Is it possible that moderate exercise affects the immune system to the point that it might even influence cancer?" asks James Rippe, M.D., director of the Exercise Physiology and Nutrition Laboratory at the University of Massachusetts.

The answer: No one knows, but scientists are investigating. Several studies have found that higher levels of fitness and exercise are correlated with lower rates of colon and breast cancer. "It's been argued that people who exercise regularly have more regular bowel movements, so they get rid of carcinogens more promptly," Dr. Rippe points out. "Or that both breast and colon cancer are associated with higher levels of body fat, which are often reduced by exercise, possibly lowering the likelihood of both those cancers."

But Dr. Rippe believes there may be something more. "I think it's also possible that there's a yet-to-be-discovered link between fitness and the immune system, a link that in some way is protecting people who are fit to some degree from getting malignancies."

Other scientists argue that even though changes in the immune system from exercise are temporary, it's still possible that they may help beat back cancer-infected cells. John Morley, M.D., professor of medicine at St. Louis University, says, "Think of tumor cells forming and escaping into the bloodstream, looking for a place to land. While they're trying to choose the ideal place to settle down, exercise triggers a sudden but temporary burst of immune cells that come out and overwhelm the tumor cells—that's a possible scenario." At this early stage of research, scientists aren't convinced that exercise reduces cancer risk by influencing the immune system. But whether there's an immune connection or not, researchers are able to say with increasing certainty that moderate regular exercise is linked to longevity and reduced cancer risk.

Walking toward Wellness

The scientists consulted by *Prevention* agreed: Walking—perhaps already America's favorite form of moderate exercise—is a safe and pleasant way to become fitter and possibly to enhance immunity. It's challenging enough to give the immune system at least a temporary boost but, done within reason, not exhausting enough to overstress the system.

Each individual should find the workout level that's comfortable for them, says Dr. Tomasi, and fitness should be built up slowly and gradually.

The scientists also warn: Don't try to maintain your walking schedule if you have a fever or infection. Exercise can spread infection throughout the body, and the immune system is already working to full capacity. Talk to your doctor if you're in doubt about exercising with an illness.

Foods That Build Your Natural Defense System

Your immune system not only determines how well you cope with cuts and colds; it can also prevent and control more serious ailments, like cancer. Aquired immune deficiency syndrome (AIDS) is so destructive because it knocks out the immune system, leaving its victims vulnerable to a host of different infections.

Unfortunately, science hasn't yet perfected drugs that strengthen human immunity. That's why scientists are investigating other ways to influence the system, including nutrition.

"It appears that one way we can modify immune function is through diet," asserts Jeffrey Blumberg, Ph.D., associate director of the U.S. Department of Agriculture's Human Nutrition Research Center on Aging, at Tufts University, Boston. "And, more important, we're finding that there are specific nutrients associated with controlling the immune system."

The link between nutrition and immunity was first noted more than 40 years ago. Physicians in developing countries observed that malnourished children suffered more infections than those who were adequately nourished.

"Now, we're beginning to learn that certain nutrients seem to be very important for one kind of immune cell and not for another," says Johns Hopkins immunologist William Beisel, M.D. "So it's becoming evident we have to understand how each nutrient works and why the immune system needs that particular nutrient."

The immune system may be particularly sensitive to nutrient deficiencies. Imagine your immune system as a sort of magical army, in which some soldiers and scouts are on permanent duty in your bloodstream. Your "good guys" include several different types of white blood cells, each with its own special mission. Together, they work to identify the threat, rouse each other, and clone into enormous armies. The armies attack and destroy your enemies: bacteria, viruses, parasites, and fungi. The action happens so quickly that you might never know you were threatened.

"You produce billions of new cells every day; they live a few days and have to be replaced. The immune system is huge and has a high turnover of infection-fighting cells. So it may be more vulnerable to deficiencies of essential nutrients than other tissues," says Pamela Fraker, Ph.D., immunologist and professor of biochemistry at Michigan State University in East Lansing.

But that doesn't mean more is always better. Scientists have documented that nutritional excesses can slow down your internal warriors, the same way that nutritional deficiencies can.

Scientists on the front lines of this research are among the first to admit that it is in its infancy. "If you really appreciate how complex the immune system is, you know that this is a field that's still emerging," says Patricia Johnston, Ph.D., whose own work examines the impact of dietary fats on immune cells.

Beyond Standard Hospital Fare

One area where nutritional immunology is already being applied is in hospitals. Why? Because many people who are ill or injured are also undernourished.

"Usually if you think of malnutrition, you think of starving people in drought-stricken countries," says Dr. Beisel. "But it happens in hospitals, too. People who suffer life-threatening diseases or serious injuries or who undergo major surgery usually lose a great deal of weight. A lot of their body nutrients are lost also. So, in our most modern medical centers, the sickest patients are very often in a state of malnutrition.

"Malnourished people are susceptible to all sorts of organisms, which can really seal their death warrant. The villain can be a fungus, a yeast, and/or common bacteria that wouldn't usually pose a problem to a healthy person," Dr. Beisel explains.

Physicians haven't always appreciated the importance of good nutrition to ward off infection among people who are ailing, says Adria Rothman-Sherman, Ph.D., chair of nutritional sciences at Rutgers University. "In the past, the approach following surgery, say, to the gastrointestinal tract, was to keep the patient on intravenous electrolytes (sodium, potassium, chloride) or glucose (sugars) until he or she could tolerate solid food. Now, we offer an intravenous formula that includes a full spectrum of essential nutrients. This really improves the patient's nutritional status and the ability of his immune system to defend his body against postoperative infections," says Dr. Rothman-Sherman.

Scientists say more can be done to make these formulas as immune-enhancing as possible. At the Shriners' Burns Institute in Cincinnati, Ohio, registered dietitian Michele Gottschlich, Ph.D., and J. Wesley Alexander, M.D., Sc.D., have found that they can reduce infection rates among burn patients with a special diet.

"Most of the standard formulas for burn patients are high in fat and linoleic acid [a polyunsaturated vegetable oil] and low in protein," explains Dr. Gottschlich. "But we're finding that too much fat can suppress immunity. And it's not just quantity of fat, but also the type of fat that has an impact on immune competence. Fish oil appears to be most beneficial. It also appears that vitamins A, C, and zinc help boost the immune response. When we combined all these elements in one formula, we significantly improved the patients' outcomes."

Of the 60 patients who participated in the study, those taking the Shriners' formula recovered better than those taking the standard formula. They had significantly fewer infections, a major complication with burn victims. And they stayed in the hospital for a shorter time. "We feel comfortable linking these results to the immune system," says Dr. Gottschlich, although specific immune-cell changes in the patients' blood were not tracked.

Immunity, Aging, and Vitamin E

Scientists at the U.S. Department of Agriculture's Human Nutrition Research Center on Aging, at Tufts University, have raised a similarly tantalizing possibility. Their research suggests that better nutrition might slow the decline in immunity that occurs with aging.

With age, Dr. Blumberg explains, there are many changes in the immune system. T-cells and B-cells (two types of white blood cell) are not as lively, for example. "We assume that these changes are at least partially responsible for the increased rate of diseases among older people: infectious diseases, cancer, and what we call the 'prolonged postillness recovery period.' That's when your body doesn't spring back after an illness as quickly as it did when you were younger."

This decline, says Dr. Blumberg, happens to everyone to a greater or lesser degree, "though the variability is tremendous between people. We don't understand why, but I'd suggest two obvious reasons. One is genetics. And the other is diet."

As people get older, many don't eat as well as they should. The elderly often lose their appetite, or they take medications that can alter appetite or impair the body's ability to absorb key nutrients. All of these factors may take a toll on their immune system, says Dr. Blumberg. This makes the natural immune decline of aging even worse.

Nutritionists agree that it's important for the elderly to eat well to avoid or reverse deficiency-related problems. But the Tufts researchers have gone one step further. Their research suggests that even among healthy and "well-nourished" elderly, vitamin E supplementation can actually make the immune system "younger."

Dr. Blumberg, along with Simin Nikbin Meydani,

D.V.M., Ph.D., and their colleagues, began their work on nutritional immunology with animal studies.

"We measured a variety of parameters of immune function in animals that were deficient in vitamin E, sufficient, or supplemented with high levels," Dr. Blumberg explains. "Although the results were complex, by and large we saw significant improvements in immunity with vitamin E supplementation."

To determine how vitamin E might have brought about this improvement, the researchers then took a closer look at the chemicals released by the immune cells. "One of these chemicals is prostaglandin E, which is an inhibitor of immune function," says Dr. Blumberg. "Immune cells need inhibitors to turn them off when they're done fighting the threat. But we found that as animals got older, they produced more and more prostaglandin E. That means more inhibiting effects on the immune system.

"We found that vitamin E supplementation reduced the production of prostaglandin E. In other words, vitamin E seems to turn off the off switch. The result is that the immune system is turned on." Dr. Blumberg and his colleagues also found that amounts of another important substance, interleukin 2, a T-cell growth factor, increased with vitamin E supplementation.

"The results of the animal tests were dramatic. And since vitamin E is one of those nutrients that is quite safe, we decided to begin human trials right away," says Dr. Blumberg.

In his study, 32 healthy volunteers, age 60 and over, came to live at the center for over a month. They were put on a carefully controlled, nutritionally balanced diet that included the U.S. Recommended Daily Allowance (US-RDA) for vitamin E. Half were given vitamin E supplementation—800 international units daily for 30 days—and the other half received a placebo (inactive substance). Neither the volunteers nor the researchers knew which capsule they were taking.

To test the patients' immune response, researchers conducted skin and blood tests. First, they injected a mild irritant into the patient's skin and measured swelling, which indicates the activity of immune cells. Next, they took blood samples and, in a test tube, exposed the blood to foreign challengers, to test the blood cell response.

Results? "In the placebo group, about 40 percent improved in immune function, 40 percent became worse, and 20 percent had no change," says Dr. Blumberg. But in the vitamin E-supplemented group, "80 percent of the people showed significant improvement."

Dr. Blumberg and other scientists caution, however, that while these results are exciting, they don't constitute final scientific proof. "To convincingly demonstrate an association between nutrition and immune function, you'd have to follow along the elderly and relate changes in their immune status to adverse outcomes, like increased urinary tract infections, skin infections or pneumonia. Then you'd have to show that by giving specific nutrients you can reverse those outcomes," says immunologist Robert Edelman, M.D.

Dr. Blumberg agrees. "It's a leap of faith to say that your risk of disease will be less if you take vitamin E."

There's no question, more work needs to be done; further studies are planned. But, so far, the Tufts researchers are very excited about the prospects. "It's worth noting that this study was conducted on normal, healthy elderly, not on those who were frail and vitamin E deficient," says Dr. Blumberg. "And yet we were still able to improve—to optimize, if you will—their immunity; to get their immune system to show the kind of responsiveness that you would expect in a really vigorous system." Keep in mind, too, that the potential applications of this research are not limited to the elderly. We know the immune decline begins after puberty, says Dr. Blumberg. So the immune-building power of good nutrition may have direct relevance to at least everybody over the age of 12 or so.

Nutrition and AIDS

Like age-related immune decline, the progression of AIDS, an immune-deficiency disease, is widely variable.

It's difficult to predict who will progress rapidly and who will progress slowly. So, here again, scientists are asking the question: Could diet be a contributing factor?

A pioneering researcher in the field, Ranjit K. Chandra, M.D., has observed that the changes in immune function in AIDS patients are very similar to those observed in malnourished people in developing countries.

Scientists are now trying to determine exactly which nutrient deficiencies AIDS patients are likely to experience. They hope their findings provide clues to an immune-strengthening diet. At a recent New York Academy of Sciences conference on nutrition and immunity, John Bogden, Ph.D., presented a study on nutritional deficiency among 30 people who tested positive for the AIDS virus. These people were at various stages of the disease; 6 were carriers with no overt symptoms, 17 had AIDS-related complex (a mild form of the disease), and 7 had AIDS.

Dr. Bogden found that 87 percent of the subjects had at least one abnormally low blood level of vitamins and trace elements, including zinc, calcium, magnesium, choline, and ascorbate (a form of vitamin C). "The number of abnormally low results substantially exceeds what we'd expect in a normal population," says Dr. Bogden. "At least we can pinpoint which nutrients are low."

The researchers don't know whether the deficiencies are the result of the virus itself or other related factors. (AIDS patients can become so ill they can't eat properly.) "Whatever the cause, malnutrition could compromise an AIDS patient's ability to combat infection," says Dr. Bogden.

Research on nutrition and AIDS is obviously in the early stages. "So far, no researchers in this area have proved they can prolong life," comments Dr. Edelman. "But AIDS patients who eat well feel better than those who consume a less-than-adequate diet." Some say, for now, that's reason enough to make good nutrition a high priority in AIDS treatment.

Helping People Get Well

"I think doctors need to consider more carefully the kind of nutrition they provide their patients, taking into account each individual's health problem. We're still giving everybody in hospitals the same food or IV (intravenous) formulas," says Dr. Fraker.

Eventually, we may see diets tailored to different illnesses. "In the future, maybe we'll know which diseases cause an increased demand for certain nutrients. Then we can replace the appropriate nutrients necessary to improve a patient's chances of survival," says Dr. Beisel.

Meanwhile, there are lessons here each of us can put into practice right away.

"Any infection alters metabolism and increases our needs for most nutrients," says Dr. Chandra. So, if you're ill, let your appetite be your guide for just a few days. Then be sure to eat lots of nutritious foods, even if you don't feel particularly hungry.

Likewise, if you're planning to undergo elective surgery, "you want to be in optimal health going into stressful surgery," says Dr. Rothman-Sherman.

The Bottom Line

And what's the best diet for those of us who want to stay healthy?

Not surprisingly, the consensus among the experts is the diet that *Prevention* has been advocating for some time.

"I suggest eating a diet low in fats, rich in complex carbohydrates, like whole grains, fruits, and vegetables," says Dr. Rothman-Sherman. "For iron and zinc, the most reliable and best sources are red meats; I suggest eating lean meat in moderate amounts."

The other scientists agree. Reduce excess fat intake. Aim for five to six servings of fruits and vegetables per day, especially red and yellow vegetables and fruits that are high in beta-carotene and vitamin C; and two servings of fish per week.

And what about supplements?

The experts' opinions differed slightly, although everyone stressed moderation. The overriding concern among nutritional immunologists is that too much supplementation of certain nutrients, especially vitamins A and B_6, iron, zinc, and selenium, can harm immunity or be toxic.

"In some cases, it's possible that a little higher than RDA [Recommended Dietary Allowance] levels may improve immune responsiveness, but higher than those levels, you're in the range of toxicity," says Dr. Blumberg.

"I personally tell people to take a multivitamin tablet a day. I think moderate doses will not harm, and will possibly help," Dr. Edelman notes.

Dr. Rothman-Sherman has a more conservative view. "I wouldn't suggest taking supplements unless there's reason to believe you're at risk of deficiency. That is, if you're on a very low-calorie diet, on medication, pregnant or lactating, or recovering from severe illness.

"If someone chooses to take a supplement," she adds, "my caution would be to supplement moderately, right around the RDA, particularly with iron. There is literature that suggests too much iron is devastating to the immune system."

Dr. Blumberg draws a distinction between vitamin E and other nutrients.

"Our studies suggest that, while most Americans get enough vitamin E to prevent a deficiency, they are not getting enough in their diets to optimize immune response. Intake would have to be higher than the current RDA of 15 to 30 international units. How much higher? I don't know. But we may need to take supplements to reach the optimal level."

Keep in mind, however, that while vitamin E is generally considered nontoxic in doses as high as 1,200 international units per day, that's not to say it's perfectly safe for you. Mild side effects, such as nausea, diarrhea, rapid pulse, itchy rash, headache, extreme fatigue, muscle weakness, and blurred vision, have been noted with doses higher than 400 international units a day. More important, vitamin E can interact with various medications. It can cause bleeding in persons taking anticlotting drugs, for example. Check with your physician if you have an existing health problem before supplementing with vitamin E.

You should not consider vitamin E supplementation as a substitute for a good diet.

The Best Defenders

Today's research in nutritional immunology involves sorting out the immune-enhancing—and sometimes, with excessive supplementation, immune-suppressing—effects of various nutrients. Until we learn more, remember: You can't overdose on nutrients in healthy foods. Choose from the list of foods below. According to the latest research, they're among your best (and safest) bets to boost immunity.

Vitamin A and the Carotenoids • Protect against tumor growth, possibly by boosting white blood cell activity. Deficiency results in overall decrease in immune function. Excess supplementation with vitamin A is toxic. Vitamin A is available in liver. Carotenoids are available in most vegetables and fruits, especially those with orange flesh, such as carrots, sweet potatoes, and cantaloupe.

Vitamin B$_6$ • Aids in metabolism of amino acids and DNA. Excess supplementation is toxic. It's available in whole grains, dark green leafy vegetables, potatoes, nuts, meats, and poultry.

Folate • Deficiency results in overall decrease in immune function. Folate is available in dark green leafy vegetables, eggs, legumes, liver, and salmon.

Vitamin C • May help strengthen the immune system's first line of defense. It's available in broccoli, sweet peppers, black currants, turnip greens, kale, and brussels sprouts, as well as in citrus and other fruits, such as berries and melons.

Vitamin E • Affects the immune system at several levels. Prevents oxidative damage to cells. Improves white blood cell activity. Vitamin E is available in wheat germ, whole grains, and vegetable oils.

Iron • Deficiency appears to raise susceptibility to infection. But infection flare-ups have been observed when iron is added to intravenous formulas. Excess supplementation is toxic. It's available in meats and poultry, eggs, dark green leafy vegetables, raisins, and whole grains.

Selenium • Prevents oxidative damage to cells. Deficiency is rare in humans. Excess supplementation is toxic. Selenium is available in seafoods, meats, poultry, eggs, whole grains, and garlic.

Zinc • Affects immunity at several levels. Deficiency results in decreased white blood cell activity. Excess supplementation is toxic. It's available in whole grains, milk, oats, oysters, eggs, meat, and poultry.

Omega-3 Fatty Acids • Appear to increase white blood cell activity. Available in salmon, mackerel, trout, and other fish.

Shape Up
for Health

Outpacing Illness

A good bet for the out-of-shape and overweight, walking is a preventive health measure of the highest order. But for some, walking offers even more; it's a path to recovery, a prescription for healing. And no one can appreciate it more than those who've literally walked away from major illness. Their unanimous call: "If we can do it, so can you!"—with the your doctor's okay.

Beating Diabetes

Watching Walter Stein lead a pack of robust racewalkers toward the finish line, you'd have to be moved. Only a year or so ago, the Monmouth County, New Jersey, Democratic committeeman collapsed in his office in a diabetic coma; his blood sugar skyrocketed to 700 (80 to 120 is normal). Back then, Stein was a self-confessed couch potato, crushing the springs at 290 pounds. His doctor laid it on the line: Keep it up, he told him, and you won't be around much longer.

"I knew I had to do something. But what?" Stein recalls. "Then I just happened to see an advertisement for a 1-mile fun walk at the New Jersey Waterfront Marathon. Even though I'd never before in my life done anything like that, I walked it."

He finished huffing and puffing. A few walks later he was hooked. Within three months he entered his first official racewalk, a 2-miler in New York's Central Park. By that time he had lost 50 pounds and his blood sugar had dropped to 250. Soon after that his doctor, Barton Nassberg, M.D., took him off all medication.

"I see a big improvement in all my diabetic patients who walk," says Dr. Nassberg. "I encourage them to walk after dinner, when blood sugar peaks. Exercising when blood sugar is low can cause dizziness in diabetics. Exercising after dinner won't have that effect. In fact, it can actually help normalize blood sugar."

His advice is right on target. Walking (with your doctor's okay) comes highly recommended by the American Diabetes Association.

Walter Stein got lots of support on his way to better health. He remembers former Olympic racewalker Elliott Denman cheering him on at the finish line during a February snowstorm. Now, it's Stein's turn to inspire others. His weight is 190 pounds, and his blood sugar is between 75 and 90.

Sidestepping Asthma

A double dose of asthma and emphysema left Leon Lewis so breathless he had to arrange his life to accommodate his lungs. The 63-year-old New York publicist would take the bus so he wouldn't have to climb the subway stairs. He'd hail a cab rather than walk a few blocks. He knew his four-pack-a-day cigarette habit was a big part of the problem. But he couldn't quit. He kept smoking even after severe asthma attacks landed him in the hospital—four times! His doctor warned him his next attack could be his last.

On a friend's suggestion, he started walking. "Just a block or two at first," says Lewis. "But slowly I was able to walk farther and farther. I began to see that smoking interfered with the 'exercise high' that I got when I walked. I really enjoyed walking, so I stopped smoking."

Soon after that, Lewis enrolled in an exercise training program for asthmatics at the Pulmonary Function Laboratory at New York University Medical Center. There, guided by director Francois Haas, Ph.D., he began walking

15-minute miles on a treadmill and doing other exercises while his breathing was monitored. His asthma attacks lessened. "For the first time in years, I felt like I could breathe freely," Lewis exclaimed.

It's not unusual for out-of-shape asthmatics to have attacks during physical exertion, says Dr. Haas. When they start to breathe heavily their bronchial tubes go into spasms. Then they really have to fight for their breath. But by conditioning the lungs—through gradually increasing activity—bronchial tubes become less reactive. This allows people with asthma to be physically active.

"Of course, anyone with asthma should consult a physician before beginning a walking program," says Dr. Haas. "If a patient's condition is stable enough for him to begin a walking program, I tell the patient to keep an inhaler on hand, and, if necessary, premedicate with albuterol or cromolyn sodium or both, 15 to 30 minutes before walking. I also instruct patients to warm up and cool down with slow walking and stretches."

Lewis started that way, walking about 20 minutes at a stretch. Now, at 73, he logs about 4 miles a day.

Helping the Heart

Ralph Riemer, 45, was working as a respiratory equipment technician at St. Mary's Hospital in Rochester, Minnesota, when he began to have chest pains. He'd had similar symptoms for a few weeks, each time he walked up a long ramp at the hospital. This time, though, the pain didn't disappear when he sat down to rest; his arms and neck started to ache, too. Riemer headed for the emergency room, where his fears were confirmed: He was having a heart attack.

Tests revealed that Riemer had two blocked arteries. Both were opened with balloon angioplasty. Then, at his doctor's behest, Riemer began doing something he'd been postponing for years: He started to exercise.

Within days of his heart attack, he was given an exercise (treadmill) stress test. A week later he started working out on a treadmill at a nearby cardiac rehabilitation center.

From there, he started walking around his neighborhood. At first, he put in about a mile a day. Eventually, he worked up to 5 miles a day, at least three times a week.

"I start everyone off walking; it's integral to our cardiac rehabilitation program," says William Freeman, M.D., Riemer's doctor at the Mayo Clinic. "Most people we see are very out of shape. So we have to ease them into exercise very slowly. Our incremental walking program, which continues for at least four to six months after the heart attack, does just that. Many patients enjoy walking so much that they continue indefinitely." The American Heart Association agrees that many heart patients can benefit from walking, as long as they have their doctor's go-ahead.

The stress test is a prerequisite to any cardiac rehab program. It shows the doctor if any heart blockages remain and how long a patient can walk without stressing his heart. In fact, regular walking offers unbeatable benefits for most hearts: It often lowers triglycerides and low-density lipoprotein (LDL) cholesterol (the "bad" kind), raises high-density lipoprotein (HDL) cholesterol (the "good" kind), improves cardiac conditioning, may help reduce blood pressure, and encourages weight loss. (Excess weight puts a strain on the heart.)

Ralph Riemer has lost 30 pounds; his cholesterol and triglyceride numbers are now in the safe range; his resting pulse rate has dropped 30 points. "It's nice to have a second chance," he says. "I haven't felt this good in years."

Outpacing Osteoporosis

Even as a young woman, Marilyn Sousa saw the effects of osteoporosis. Her mother wore an old-fashioned brace to support her weakened spine. At the time, no one knew that the immobilizing corset would make her spine weaker.

Today, decades later, Marilyn has osteoporosis, too. But instead of cutting down on the action, Marilyn has stepped hers up. She walks 2 miles every morning and 2 more every night.

She has been a patient at the Osteoporosis Center at the University of Connecticut Health Center for 15 years.

There, JoAnne Smith, M.D., and other doctors make exercise an important part of a program that includes hormone or fluoride treatment and calcium supplementation.

"The important thing is to maintain people's bone strength," Dr. Smith says. "We've found that weight-bearing exercise like walking helps to keep bones dense, just as weight-lifting helps strengthen muscles." Walking also improves muscle tone and balance; both help avoid falls.

Older women's bones may already be weak. They need to build up slowly, Dr. Smith warns. "Our patients start walking 10 minutes three to four times a week. If that goes well, they add 5 minutes a week until they are up to 45 minutes of walking per workout." Too much, too soon, can cause stress fractures, especially in the delicate bones of the feet and shins. Foot, leg, hip, or back pain is a sign to stop walking and see a doctor.

Thanks to the program at the Osteoporosis Center, Marilyn Sousa has been able to maintain her bone mass for 15 years now. Unlike her mother, who was bound in a corset, she is bounding with energy.

Rambling Relaxation

New Jersey advertising executive Robert Milo remembers staring for two days at a prescription for tranquilizers his doctor had given him. "I was under a lot of stress, but I was afraid of the addictive power of pills," he says. "I never did take one." Instead, he saw psychologist William Rosenblatt, Ed.D., at the Biofeedback and Stress Management Center in Morristown, New Jersey. There, he says, "I found the best tranquilizer ever—walking."

He pops a special relaxation tape into his portable tape deck and heads out the door. "When I'm walking, listening to music, I can feel the tension draining from my upper back and neck," he says.

"Stress triggers your body to produce adrenaline, which readies you for action," Dr. Rosenblatt explains. "If you don't take action, though, adrenaline can accumulate, causing muscle tension and feelings of anxiety."

Walking is a positive way to move you into action. It

uses up adrenaline and causes the release of calming brain chemicals called endorphins. It helps reduce tension and anxiety, according to researchers at the University of Massachusetts.

Walking also gives people a sense of control, Dr. Rosenblatt says. "When people exercise, they see that they can control (indeed, reverse) their physical reactions to stress—even if they can't control the stressful situation. As a result, they can cope better emotionally."

Work was a major headache for Robert Milo. Now his hectic day is cushioned by morning, lunchtime, and sometimes evening walks. "I'm a lot happier than I used to be!" he claims. His long laugh after that last comment lets you know he means it.

Rebounding from Back Problems

Edward Jobe lay in bed for three weeks with back pain before he finally agreed to have back surgery.

"They had me on my feet the same day as the operation," he says. The next day, he hobbled the hospital hallways; the day after that, he walked a few minutes on a treadmill. Since then, he has walked every day, frequently for an hour in the morning and a half-hour at night. He has less pain than he's had since his back problems began six years ago.

His doctor, Willibald Nagler, M.D., is a physiatrist (a doctor specializing in physical medicine and rehabilitation) at New York Hospital-Cornell University Medical Center. His pain-reduction exercise programs are used by back pain sufferers around the country.

"To have strong, aerobically trained back muscles is very important for the prevention and treatment of back pain," Dr. Nagler explains.

"It's easy enough to increase the flexibility of these muscles with stretching exercises, but increasing endurance is harder. One good way to do this is to walk, swinging your arms."

Of course, no one with a bad back should undertake a walking regimen without a doctor's okay, Dr. Nagler says.

Rest, not exercise, is best for acute back pain. And walking can worsen problems like degenerative disk disease.

For some, though, like Edward Jobe, walking can be a back saver. "I played golf on Monday and got a birdie on the 18th hole, which suggests I'm doing well," he says.

Curing Urban Ills

Sometimes, too, walking can assist ailing neighborhoods just as it can the people who live in them. How? Just ask Chett Carmichael.

Carmichael started strolling around his North Philadelphia neighborhood because he wanted to lose 50 pounds. But he soon saw that his environment was suffering from its own malaise: trash.

"I became a kind of one-man crusade," he says.

Carmichael started carrying a camera on his walks. He photographs areas of litter, truckloads of old tires under a railroad trestle, whole bags of trash in subway stations. Then he sends the photos to Philadelphia's mayor Wilson Goode, who, so far, orders city sanitation workers to the spot.

Carmichael has long since lost the 50 pounds, but his new goal keeps him hoofing 5 miles every day, each day in a different Philadelphia neighborhood. Last year he covered 900 miles.

Being committed to resolving problems that are bigger than any one person has brought new energy into Carmichael's life. He knows how having a sense of belonging can enhance health.

Glide into Shape, Climb to Higher Fitness

Experts agree: stair climbing and cross-country skiing are among the best muscle-toning, heart-pumping, feel-good-afterward workouts ever devised. Which means they're aerobic. Really aerobic. Minute for minute, they can probably do more good for your cardiovascular system than jogging can. So it was only a matter of time before they left the snowfields and the stairwells and got mechanized so you could do them anywhere, anytime, at your own calibrated pace.

One of the claims to fame for cross-country ski machines and stair climbers is their enormous calorie-burning potential. So they can help give you fast weight-loss results.

A standard 30-minute workout on either of them, done just three times a week, can burn off 2,000 calories. Such a regimen—along with cutting out 1 tablespoon of butter a day and trading in a daily glass of whole milk for a low-fat one—could help you lose 1 pound a week.

Plus, exercising on skiers and climbers gives you a no-impact workout—your joints and knees won't take a pounding as they might in jogging. And the risk of muscle strain is minimal, much lower than in, say, cycling or weight training.

With the skiers you swing your arms and legs just as you would if you were skiing across level snow, gliding smoothly and rhythmically against preadjusted resistance. It's this vigorous movement of all your limbs that provides the tremendous aerobic effect. And all major muscle groups get a good workout. It may take a few minutes of practice to get the hang of it, but anyone can do it.

The stair climbers are easier still. You just get on and go, raising your feet up and down on the movable "steps" yet staying in one spot. The big calorie-burning, oxygen-moving effect comes from rhythmically lifting your entire body weight vertically against gravity.

So both the skiers and the climbers are good bets for those who want an intense workout in a relatively short time. Or those who want a vigorous change of pace from their usual exercise routine.

If you've been working out regularly, you're ready to graduate to a skier or climber. If you've been sedentary, start with another form of exercise—walking, for instance—to develop some stamina. Keep at it for a few weeks, then try skiers or climbers.

Ski Easy, Ski Well

Cross-country ski machines sport loads of variations. The foot mechanisms may include skilike slats or cushioned pads. Your arms may get their workout with rope-and-pulley systems, or maybe poles. Some machines are bare-bones stripped-down versions (which may cost about $400). And some are high-tech, capable of recording your time, distance, and miles per hour (and cost about $600). (As with any exercise machine, it's always best to try it out at a gym or spa before buying one for yourself.)

Whatever type you kick and glide on, there are a few tricks to getting a top workout.

Loosen Up Your Ankles First • Before each workout, sit down and draw 20 clockwise circles in the air with your toes, bending at the ankles. Then 20 counterclockwise ones. How often do you ask your ankles to flex as far and as hard as they do when you're skiing? Give them a chance to get used to the idea by loosening them up first.

Learn to Properly Shift Your Weight as You Stride • This is the number one requirement for an effective and safe skier workout. The idea is to shift your weight over the ball of the foot that's starting a backward kick, then shift weight to the other side just as that foot glides forward under your body. When you don't shift your weight and just slide the skis back and forth, you're doing the "cheater's shuffle."

Your feet will give you away—they'll start lifting out of the toe clips or footpads.

Practice the leg movements first, then the arm movements. If you're just learning how to use a skier, ignore the arm mechanism for now and focus on the kick-glide. Hang on to the hip bumper or handrails for balance. Or try keeping your arms at your sides and swinging them as you would when walking. When you've got the kick-glide down pat, then integrate the arm swinging.

Stand Erect and Keep Your Eyes Straight Ahead • Watching your feet and hunching over the hip bumper will give you a curled-over posture—which undoes some of the benefits of the workout. The opportunity to exercise upright (on the skier or stair climber) is a big advantage for desk jockeys and others who spend their days sedentary and hunched over. You can almost hear the "Ahhhhhhhh" of relief as you stretch and extend your lower back muscles.

Hold the Bumper Pad Firmly to Your Abdomen with Your Hands • That protects your lower back by stopping the pelvic rotation caused by kicking your legs back—an invitation to backache. Adjust the pad so that it rides low on your pelvis, but not so low as to interfere with your thigh coming forward. If you still have back trouble after a workout, get some back-strengthening exercises from an expert, maybe a trainer at your local health club. Of course, if you've had medical treatment for your back, ask your doctor for advice.

Maintain Your Equipment • If you're exercising on your own skier, it pays to oil the arm and leg mechanisms occasionally and to wipe the shoe grit off the rails. Well-lubricated, dirt-free rails and gears ensure that you'll always have a smooth, bump-free workout.

Adjusting Your Heart for Skiing or Climbing

You get the most out of any aerobic exercise when your heart thumps away at an increased but safe speed—what's called your "target heart rate." That's usually about 75 to 80 percent of your maximum safe heart rate. But for workouts on ski machines and stair climbers, your target rate should be about 60 percent of maximum. It's just too easy to start working too hard on these machines, overstressing heart and lungs. Besides, if you start sweating heavily too early in your workout, your muscles will fatigue and you won't last long enough to enjoy serious fat-searing results.

To figure your 60-percent-of-maximum target rate, subtract your age from 220. Multiply that number by 0.6. During workouts, periodically take your pulse or use a small heart monitor to check your progress.

Stepping Up to Shapeliness

These days just about all stair climbers are computerized, and some let you program different warm-up, workout, and cool-down sessions. Some models function by depressing two paddles with your feet. Some let you climb up a "down" escalator. Climbers start at about $450; a top-of-the-line climber costs about $2,500.

Whatever type you use, follow these rules of climbing for maximum results.

Rest Your Hands Lightly on the Rails • Do this for balance only. Firmly clutching the handrails transfers some of your weight to your arms. But the weight's got to be on your legs to guarantee the maximum fat burn from your workout. If you have to hang on to the handrails to keep up the pace, you're going too fast.

Make Sure Your Knees Move Forward, Staying over Your Toes • If you place your foot ahead of your knee and then try to lift up on that foot, your knee may get strained. Which is not to say stair climbing is hazardous to knees when it's done properly.

On Programmable Models, Customize Your Workout Time • Many people who use a climber assume that they're stuck with the workout the climber's computer has programmed for them—usually 15 minutes long. They think that to get a minimum 20-minute workout, they have to stop, reset the machine for another 15 minutes, then stop it again after 5. But you can program the climber to go for 20 minutes—just check your owner's manual or ask your health-club attendant for help.

Try "Muscle-Specific" Workouts • You can actually design your climbing to tone certain muscles, like those in your behind. Just take higher steps, letting the machine carry your foot farther down. And to work on those abdominal muscles, take shorter steps, keeping your feet a little forward of your upper torso.

Mini Motivators

Whether you go with skier or climber, there are a few gadgets and gimmicks that can help you keep at it.

Check your form in a mirror. Watch your upright stance on a skier, monitor your knee-toe alignment on a climber, or just admire your ever-shapelier self with a wall-mounted mirror.

Add some motivational posters, if they reflect your true convictions. Some "Rome wasn't built in a day"-type posters may help you keep gliding and climbing, week after week. Hang them near the machine where you can't possibly miss them.

Let the sun shine in—but not on—your workout. Sunshine will brighten up your workout area—and probably your workout. But don't overdo it. Placing your machines directly in the sun's rays can turn you into a solar-heat collector.

Try a portable heart rate monitor. A pulse monitor that clips to your ear or finger costs $60 to $150; a heart monitor goes for about $150 to $300. Ask at a sporting-goods store. A monitor makes it easy to check your exertion level at a glance and gives you I-can-do-it incentive.

Position your exercise equipment in the coolest spot in your house. A room that's comfortable for lounging may seem like a sauna while you're skiing or climbing. Temperatures in the low 60s are best.

Choose the right music. Listening to music can motivate you, but a too-dominant rock-type beat can compete with the steady pace you're striving to maintain. Try show tunes or the "Brandenburg Concertos" instead.

Row and Ride
to a Better Body

No pain, no rain. No wind or ice or gloom of early winter nights to keep you from your appointed rounds of exercise.

That's the big appeal of indoor cycling and rowing. With no excuses, they're the easiest, surest exercise methods to slim down. To give your heart a bracing but safe workout. To dissolve the day's accumulation of stress.

Because bikes and rowing machines support your weight, you may be able to use them even if you can't do other exercises. If your knees or hamstrings are feeling the result of too much running, these machines can save your fitness program. And they can be especially valuable for people with moderate arthritis.

Biking or rowing, like any exercise, helps you look better and lose weight by burning off extra fat, improving muscle tone, and dampening your appetite. By combining biking or rowing with a sensible diet, you can safely lose 1 to 2 pounds a week. For example, if you were to row or cycle at moderate intensity for 30 minutes a day during a week (six days of workouts, one day of rest), you'd burn 900 calories (150 calories per workout). And if, during that same week, you cut your calorie intake by about 300 calories a day, you'd be getting rid of another 2,100 calories or so. Between the exercise and the dieting, you can lose nearly a pound a week.

Just see your doctor before jumping into such a regimen. He can make sure you're ready to start and help you with diet and behavior to maximize weight loss.

Starting a New Cycle

If you're gearing up for weight loss through stationary biking, here's how to get the most mileage from the experience.

Make Sure Your Bike Fits • If it doesn't, you won't feel comfortable. In fact, you could hurt yourself. Start with the saddle—women's biggest complaint about bikes. Check the width by sitting on it. The saddle should support your pelvic bones, not dig into your flesh. If the saddle does dig into you, have a bike dealer show you some wider ones. If you're using a gym bike and can't readily change the seat, cushion it with a foam or sheepskin pad.

Then check saddle height. If you push the pedal all the way down with the ball of your foot, your knee should be slightly flexed.

Next, adjust the cant—the angle of the saddle. (Even on the cheapest of bikes you should be able to adjust the seat.) If the front is too high, it can cause discomfort. Remedy: Adjust the saddle so the front is parallel to the top tube or tipped slightly down.

Once the seat is right, check the handlebar. Set the height and angle so, when you hold it, you lean only slightly forward. Place just a little weight on your arms. That way, you're not likely to strain your lower back.

Take It Easy, Especially at First • Set the bike's resistance low enough that you can pedal comfortably. Too much resistance can inflame tendons and hurt ligaments and cartilage in your knee.

A good beginner's workout goes like this: First do 40 revolutions per minute (rpm)—10 revolutions every 15 seconds—for 3 to 5 minutes. Then move to the main part of the workout. Accelerate to 60 rpm: 1 revolution per second. An easy way to estimate this is to count "one thousand one, one thousand two . . ." with each revolution. Try to keep cycling for a total of 20 minutes.

When you've done your time, cool down by pedaling at a lower speed and resistance for 3 to 5 minutes. For your last minute, slow to 40 rpm.

You may need to modify the intensity of this regimen, of course, to maintain your target heart rate or to ensure comfort (see below). In any event, you should end this workout after the 20 to 25 minutes are up or you feel you've done enough, whichever comes first.

When you do finish, walk around the room a few minutes. And don't shower or bathe for at least 10 minutes after you stop exercising. You may unduly stress your heart.

Change Hand Positions during Workouts • Doing so changes the position of your back and arms, reducing soreness. Periodically stand up and pedal 30 seconds, too. This relieves saddle pressure and stretches your legs.

When the beginner's routine doesn't tire you, try tougher workouts. Within a few weeks, you can raise your sights to at least 70 percent, but no more than 80 percent, of your maximum heart rate. Get there by adding more resistance, riding for at least 2 minutes and checking your pulse.

Keep adjusting resistance until you can stay at your new target heart rate for a 20- to 25-minute workout. By adding 1 to 2 minutes to every other session, you can eventually work up to 45 minutes a day, six days a week.

On the seventh day, rest. Cycling six days a week is enough.

Make Sure the Bike Has a Weighted Flywheel • That's the smooth-running wheel with a friction belt that regulates resistance. Bikes that regulate resistance by increasing pressure on the wheel, or those with caliper brakes, tend to be jerky and no fun to pedal.

Get Your Money's Worth • For a decent new stationary bike with basic features, expect to pay $125 to $500. High-tech bikes cost more: $1,200 to $2,100. Some of them have displays that estimate the calories you burn, count your rpms, take you through a preprogrammed warm-up and cool-down, and let you race against a computer-generated opponent.

Try Variations • Some bikes exercise not just your legs but your arms and torso, too. As you pedal, you move the swinging handlebar back and forth with your arms. With such dual-action bikes, air resistance generates the workload, so in these models no flywheel is necessary. And, in most models, the resistance stirs the air enough to give you a pleasant breeze. If your legs get tired, you can pedal less and let your arms do the work. Price: $400 to $700.

If, because of hip or back problems, you can't use a standard indoor bicycle, you may still be able to cycle. On a recumbent exercise bike, you pedal sitting, as if you were in a chair. There's a backrest to support you, and your legs go in front of rather than underneath you. Prices start at $200.

If you have back trouble, check with your doctor before you try either the dual-action or recumbent models. And don't use them if they hurt!

Row, Row, Row to a Better Body

Like dual-action bikes, rowing machines shape up not just leg muscles but also the chest, back, trunk, and arms. Here's how to get the maximum benefits from any rowing machine.

Get Expert Help • Start your rowing career with a back evaluation, preferably from your family doctor or back specialist. He or she can prescribe exercises to stretch and strengthen your lower back muscles. Have an instructor show you proper rowing technique, too. It's easy to learn.

Adjust the Footrest to a Comfortable Angle • Otherwise, the footrest can flex your ankles uncomfortably and prevent you from making a full stroke.

Use the "Comfort Lover's" Training Schedule • To prevent back injury, begin your rowing regimen with low resistance and a minimum number of strokes. If you have arthritis, start with 20 strokes a day. Add 20 strokes a week, building up to 100. Use rowing as part of an overall fitness program.

If you don't have arthritis, warm up by rowing 12 strokes a minute for 5 minutes. Since rowing works out all the major muscle groups, you may tire quickly. Don't feel badly if the warm-up is all you can do at first. Let your heart rate, or what feels comfortable, guide you. Increase your rowing gradually, adding 10 percent a week to your number of strokes per minute. Ultimately, aim for 22 to 24 strokes per minute. When you can row for 20 minutes, add more power to your workouts. Every 2 or 3 minutes, for instance, pull harder for 10 strokes. Or alternate periods of hard rowing with easy rowing. Later, increase the time and intensity of your workout still more. And at the end of each workout, cool down with some slow stretching.

Buy Quality • Avoid rowing machines that use a knob tightened on a wheel to provide resistance. Such machines are too jerky. Two types of units are worth considering.

Hydraulic cylinder rowers, quiet and small enough to sit in a corner, are the most popular at-home models. The higher on the rowing arm you clamp the cylinder, the greater the resistance. Price: $129 to $400.

Straight-pull rowers cost more. Some come with an electronic speedometer, stroke counter, timer, calorie counter, and, like the high-tech bikes, a computer-generated rower you can race against. A flywheel braked by a fan, belt, or motor provides resistance. Price: $650 and up.

Whatever machine you buy, make sure the seat rides on ball bearings, not plastic. And look for joints that are welded together, not bolted. Bolts and plastic wear out quickly.

Good Advice for Both Bikers and Rowers

Follow your heart—or how you feel. Depending on your temperament, let one of two indicators guide the intensity of your workout. If you'd like an objective measure of how hard to cycle or row, go by your heart rate. You can estimate your maximum heart rate by subtracting your

---

Race Away from the Blahs

The biggest challenge of indoor exercise is boredom. But you can beat it.

Get a reading-rack attachment for your bike and stock it with big-print magazines and books—so you can read without leaning too far forward. Reading while rowing doesn't work, though, because of the sliding seat. On either a bike or rower you can watch television. Work out to your favorite shows, or, to simulate outdoor conditions, to videos with intriguing destinations.

Music, like video, is ready whenever you are. If you play something peppy, you can pedal or stroke to the beat.

If you need to think things out, do it on your machine. Exercise may dissipate whatever stress you feel. Or simply let your thoughts drift. Rowing and biking are fine media for meditation.

There's a physical side to beating boredom, too. Once you're in better shape, after three months or so, vary your workout with short, high-intensity bursts. Climb a hill: Increase the resistance for 60 to 90 seconds and hold your speed constant. Or imagine yourself in a race. To sprint, keep the speed constant but increase resistance above your usual level.

Should all else fail, try exercising first thing in the morning. If you work out before you're fully awake, you may not be alert enough to feel bored!

age from 220. When you exercise, you should reach 50 to 70 percent of that rate initially, and eventually work up to 75 to 80 percent. You'll probably have to slow down a bit to check your pulse. Don't slow down for long, though. Take your pulse on the artery that runs along your right wrist toward your thumb. Using the fingertips of your left hand, you should find your pulse easily. To estimate your heart rate, take your pulse for 10 seconds and multiply by six.

If you don't want to bother with the numbers, you can simply do what feels comfortable. You should be breathing deeply and rapidly, as if you've climbed a flight of stairs. But you should always have enough breath to talk while you exercise. (As in any exercise, if you feel abnormal heartbeats, pain, dizziness, or other distress, you should stop the workout and see a doctor.)

Use a fan, or fan yourself with a "wind-load" bike or rowing machine. The breeze simulates conditions outdoors, drying perspiration before it builds up too much. A fan can double the time you spend working out.

Going for the Burn

Calories burned by a 150-pound person in 30 minutes of high-intensity:

- Rowing (vigorously): 328
- Stationary cycling (15 mph, resistance sufficient to get heart rate to 130): 328
- Judo: 395
- Handball (2 people): 383
- Running (7 mph): 350
- Aerobic dancing: 328
- Jogging (5½ mph): 328
- Walking (5½ mph): 328

From *Maximum Personal Energy* by Charles T. Kuntzleman, Ed.D. (Rodale Press, 1981).

Drink water before, during, and after each session. That can help prevent dehydration and heat stress. Heat makes you tire faster, and dehydration can be dangerous.

Put your exercise machine someplace conspicuous. If it's in your living room, you're more likely to stick to your regimen than if the machine's tucked away somewhere.

Pick a workout time when you normally don't have conflicting duties. That way, excuses for skipping a workout will be just about impossible to find.

Lose Weight, Beat Diabetes

The popular concept is that diabetes is controlled with insulin injections and careful monitoring of diet (which it is, for about one million people with diabetes). But weight loss is the most effective way to prevent and treat the most common form of the disease, known as Type II or non-insulin-dependent diabetes, which affects about ten millon Americans—half of whom are unaware of their condition.

Left untreated, complications from diabetes can be fatal—leading to heart disease, stroke, and kidney failure. The nation's fourth largest killer (after heart disease, cancer, and stroke) can also lead to blindness, nerve destruction, gangrene, and blood vessel damage that can lead to amputation.

Type II diabetes generally strikes after age 40 in those who are overweight. Other factors include a family history of diabetes, or in women, having given birth to a baby weighing more than nine pounds. Although it may present no warning, typical symptoms include an unusual hunger and/or thirst; frequent need to urinate; fatigue or drowsiness; a slow-healing wound; blurred or a change in vision; frequent infection of the gums, skin, or urinary tract; intense itching; and pain or tingling in the legs or feet.

"Many Type II diabetic patients are 30 to 60 pounds

overweight," says Robert Henry, M.D., a diabetes weight-loss specialist. "For some, there's no question that losing just 10 pounds can make a big difference." With weight loss, all three major defects of Type II diabetes improve: High insulin levels drop; the liver, which has been secreting two to three times more sugar than normal into the blood, begins to produce less; and peripheral muscle tissues, previously resistant to the effect of insulin to enhance sugar uptake, now take up sugar better.

Type II diabetic individuals who take additional insulin without trying to lose weight can actually *gain* weight. That's because the insulin causes the body to store excess sugar as body fat—and too much body fat worsens diabetes. If you must take medication but can still lose a few pounds, you may be able to cut back on your dosage gradually, with medical supervision. Try these strategies to make weight loss easier.

Beware of "Diabetic" Foods • Foods labeled "dietetic" or "diabetic" can be deceptive. It's true that they contain no sugar: They contain sorbitol, a lower-calorie sugar alcohol. But some of these products are higher in fat and calories than their nondiabetic counterparts.

When It Comes to Sweets, Know Thyself • Some people with diabetes profess a strong urge for sweets, an urge only made *worse* by total denial. Nutritionists offer this solution: If you know it's going to lead to bingeing, don't try to deprive yourself of sweets totally. Instead, incorporate controlled portions of sweets into your daily diet. Others, though, know they do better if they cut out all sweets except fruits. Why? Because they "can't eat just one." It's actually *easier* for them to go cold turkey.

Plan a Snack for Your Hungriest Time • Around 4:00 P.M., the resistance of many would-be diabetic dieters drops to its lowest as their insulin level peaks. (Insulin is a well-known appetite stimulant.) This afternoon peak usually happens with naturally produced insulin (depending on when and what you've eaten so far during the day). Instead of trying to stick it out and failing, plan a snack for this or any other particularly tempting time, says Christine Beebe, R.N., who specializes in diabetes management. Take the calories from somewhere else in your day. The trick is *planning:* It protects you from impulsively eating something you'd rather not.

Avoid Weight-Loss Aids • Over-the-counter appetite suppressants that contain phenylpropanolamine (PPA) only compound the problems. They can contribute to high blood pressure and kidney and eye problems.

Learn to Check Your Blood Sugar • Monitoring blood sugar provides valuable information that can be used to adjust food or drug intake. And this monitoring is especially important in any strategy to lose weight. Some doctors lower their patients' insulin or oral insulin-stimulating drugs the day they start on a weight-loss diet. This prevents a frightening episode of low blood sugar (hypoglycemia) four or five days into the diet (which happens if blood sugar drops and insulin or oral drug dosage is still high). Most successful at losing weight, with fewest hypoglycemic episodes, are diabetics who carefully monitor their blood sugar and consult with their doctor as often as every week about having their drug dosage lowered as their blood sugar drops.

Treat Hypoglycemia without Overeating • "I'm so attuned to my physical condition that when my blood sugar drops, and I feel 'fuzzy,' I still know exactly what to eat," says Charlene Postigo, diagnosed with diabetes five years ago. She consumes precisely what will bring her blood sugar back to normal—no more. That's 4 ounces of orange or apple juice or 4 to 6 ounces of milk. To make sure it's worked, she waits 20 minutes, then tests her blood sugar. Fear of falling into a diabetic coma leads diabetics to overtreat low blood sugar with bowls of ice cream or peanut butter and jelly sandwiches. That only adds to their problems by piling on pounds.

Go High-Carb • Based on research from the past ten years or so, the American Diabetes Association (ADA) recommends a high-fiber, high-complex-carbohydrate, low-fat diet because it's been found that the fibers in whole grains and some fruits and vegetables prolong sugar absorption, stabilizing blood sugar levels. Also, by shifting away from fats, especially saturated fats, the ADA is acknowledging that cardiovascular disease is a leading cause of death among diabetes sufferers. It's also clear that complex carbohydrates (found mostly in whole grain products, beans, and vegetables) can be big pluses in any weight-loss plan. Since they're generally not calorie dense (few calories per unit of weight), you can eat a lot of them, satisfying your appetite without adding on extra pounds.

Mind/Body Healing Strategies

Can We Talk?

By Robert Ornstein, Ph.D., and
David Sobel, M.D.

You are probably quite familiar with the claim that confession is good for the soul. But confession is more than a moral issue: It can sometimes be good for the body as well. The principle is this: When there is a major trauma, it is probably healthier in the long run to face up to it. Confessing may be unpleasant at the moment, but getting it off your chest can clear your mind to enjoy a more pleasurable life.

In many lives there are extraordinary traumas, events that can scar one for life. We don't mean ordinary business disappointments, financial setbacks, or the usual marital upsets. The health-damaging secrets are the major traumas like seeing a loved one die in an accident, or witnessing a violent crime.

Men and women who had suffered the death of their spouse due to an automobile accident or suicide found that confiding is good for health. They spoke with others about their tragedies, and in the year following the death, were healthier than those who had not talked with others.

The Art of Disclosure

Although there are times when talking about upsetting things makes people more upset, encouraging people to disclose long-held traumas can measurably improve health. Psychologist James Pennebaker, Ph.D., professor of psychology at Southern Methodist University in Dallas instructed some of his students as follows: "I want you to write continuously about the most upsetting or traumatic experience of your entire life [and] discuss your deepest thoughts and feelings about the experience. Ideally, it should be about something you have not talked with others about in detail. It is critical, however, that you let yourself go and touch those deepest emotions and thoughts that you have. . . ." Meanwhile, other students simply wrote about trivial daily activities.

The students kept these diaries over four days. One student disclosed that while he was in high school he was beaten by his stepfather. Another student wrote about his feelings concerning the divorce of his parents. His father told him at age nine that he was divorcing the boy's mother because their home life had been disrupted ever since the boy had been born.

Disclosing feelings about such traumas was obviously difficult and emotionally distressing. But getting these secrets off their chest paid off in the long run. When compared to the students who wrote about something neutral like going to a ball game, the ones who confessed an emotionally traumatic event had fewer health complaints, fewer doctor visits, and fewer drugs prescribed during the following six months.

Not only undergraduate students in a psychology experiment benefit from confession. Thirty-three survivors of the Holocaust gave videotaped interviews about their experiences during World War II.

Virtually all these survivors had suffered, many of them in silence, for decades. Those who more freely described their powerful trauma reported fewer health problems.

So, confessing may be very good for the body. In the

mind, a covered-over negative event is never finished. Sometimes people tend to mull over the trauma again and again in their mind, rehearsing what they should have said, what they might have done. Writing about something or confiding in someone may force you to organize your thoughts and feelings about events, revealing hidden biases and unresolved issues. Once it's out, you may be able to distance yourself from the traumatic experience. By getting it off your chest, you may be able to break the endless cycle of negative thoughts and feelings.

This may be one of the reasons why many religious traditions, social organizations, and self-help groups encourage confession, self-disclosure, and confiding in other people. This may also help explain why people enmeshed in strong social-support networks are healthier: These networks may provide greater opportunity for people to confide their difficult experiences.

Heal Yourself the Native American Way

When patients tell their troubles to psychiatrist Carl Hammerschlag, M.D., he may suggest that they hike up a mountain. He may tell them to ponder the flight of a young eagle. He might sing them a song from the native American tradition, or even advise that they perform a ritual with their family and friends.

"Some of my colleagues think I've spent too much time in the sun," says Dr. Hammerschlag, laughing. The 50-year-old author of *The Dancing Healers: A Doctor's Journey of Healing with Native Americans* trained in psychiatry at Yale. In fact, it was his 20 years spent practicing medicine in the American Southwest that changed his vision of health and healing.

"Why people get sick, and why they get well, has to

do with the connections between mind, body, and spirit," he says. "Native Americans have always known this. Western medicine is just beginning to catch on. The new science of psychoneuroimmunology has provided us with data suggesting a link between the mind and the immune system.

"In Western medicine, doctors tend to assume most of the responsibility for making people well.

"Native American medicine men understand that the healer plays but a small role in the healing process. They tell their patients, 'I'll do the best I can. You must do the best you can. You must have faith in yourself. You must look within and call up your inner strength. You must rally the support of your family and clan. We've all got to work together.'"

Quests for Health

As a psychiatrist, Dr. Hammerschlag works primarily in the area of emotional healing. "When a person is depressed or confused, the physician's advice is just one part of the prescription for spiritual renewal. The patient needs to learn to look within to find his or her own strength," says Dr. Hammerschlag. "It's like dancing. You can't learn to dance by listening to someone explain it to you; you have to get up and do it."

That's why Dr. Hammerschlag sometimes suggests that his patients undertake tasks or "quests," inspired by native American traditions. He considers them useful lessons in what he calls the "dance of healing."

"I had a patient, a scientist, who was obsessed with perfection. When he wasn't working, he read scientific journals—even on vacations," Dr. Hammerschlag explains.

"So I told him that on his next vacation, he had to leave all his reading material behind. The only book he could take along was one that I gave him.

"What he didn't realize until he got there was that the book was full of blank pages. On the first page, however, I had written him a prescription.

"It was this: Whenever he would ordinarily read, he

was to take the empty book and go to a quiet place. There he'd open the book and allow his imagination to run wild. He could write poetry. He could draw pictures. He could find leaves and glue them on the pages. Or he could just look at the blank pages.

"Here was someone who had always tried to fill himself up from the outside," says Dr. Hammerschlag. "But the exercise helped him discover that true fulfillment comes from the inside."

Create Your Own Tasks

Dr. Hammerschlag says you can create your own tasks according to what you need to learn.

If you're sad and feeling bleak about the future, it won't make you feel any better if someone tells you not to worry, things will improve, Dr. Hammerschlag explains. You've got to experience that sense of hopefulness for yourself. To do that, he says, go to a beautiful place where you can be reminded that from darkness comes the light. Camp out on a mountaintop or walk along the seashore before daybreak.

The idea is to experience the darkness and then the light of dawn.

If you're fearful of an impending big move—changing jobs, buying a new home, going back to school, take a small, enjoyable risk. Ask yourself: What is it that I've always wanted to do? To learn to sail? To snorkle? To ski? To visit Alaska? Pick one you'll enjoy and do it. "Knowing you can succeed with the small risk will give you the strength you need to succeed with the bigger risk," Dr. Hammerschlag notes.

If your exercise routine has crossed the line between good sense and compulsion, next time, stop halfway. Take a mountain trail and stop short of the top. There, mid-mountain, find a peaceful place to sit and think. The reason: "Compulsive people only feel good if they've hit the finish line," Dr. Hammerschlag explains. "They need to understand that the end is not where they thought it was. That the end might really be in the middle."

Let Nature Be Your Guide

Dr. Hammerschlag speaks in a slow, deep, hypnotic voice, ideal for another one of his unorthodox approaches to helping people: story telling. He learned from native American healers that stories about the natural world can be powerful tools to guide people to a deeper understanding of their own lives.

If you're coping with empty-nest syndrome—that is, your children are growing up and leaving home—find solace in the story of the eagles.

"The gift we have to give our children is roots—to ground them in a good way—and wings—to allow them to fly," says Dr. Hammerschlag.

"People who are dealing with the empty-nest syndrome need to sense the fulfillment we get when we watch a young bird fly. That's why I tell them about eagles.

"Eagles mate for life. Each year, they lay a single egg. Their nests are usually in a very precarious place, on a cliff.

"There, their single most prized possession is exposed to the elements because they have faith something good will happen. The parent birds take care of it even if they have to starve themselves. The baby bird doesn't move from the nest, because it can't fly. Then, one day, it's time; the young bird takes off and flies by itself. Never in the history of eagledom has a young eagle taken off and not flown. Now, the parents can see their eagle raise other eagles. And they can watch their gift being shared with the next generation.

"This story gets people in touch with the idea that, in giving away, they get something back."

Revel in Ritual

Dr. Hammerschlag says that one of the most important lessons he has learned from the native Americans is that rituals involving family and friends can be very powerful in healing.

"In Western cultures, we don't think of ritual as a means of mind/body/spirit healing. Instead we attach our-

selves to science and technology. Science does not have all
the answers. This is not to put down the great advances of
science; if my retina becomes detached, I want someone to
reattach it with a laser.

"But most of life doesn't deal with retinal attachment;
most of it deals with ordinary ups and downs, crises, and
stressful life events, which don't lend themselves to scientific analysis."

When you face important events, happy or sad, create
a ritual that includes your family and friends. "Ritual and
ceremony can help reconnect you to the idea that you're
not alone," says Dr. Hammerschlag.

"We've always known anecdotally that if someone
cares about you, you'll deal better with whatever it is you
have to confront. One of the great failings of the pop psychological movement is the idea that everybody does it
alone; 'Do your own thing,' 'Paddle your own canoe,' 'Be
captain of your own ship.' That's nonsense."

Ceremonies can help us cope with the most difficult
situations. "I know one family who was devastated when
their child was born blind," Dr. Hammerschlag notes.
"Then they decided to give up the idealized fantasy of what
they thought the child should be, to allow the child its own
creativity and uniqueness. The family held a ceremony. All
the participants talked about their hopes for the child. They
allowed each other to express their feelings of pain and
sadness, to give up those feelings, to celebrate the child for
who she was, to offer each other support, and to get on
with business. These kinds of rituals are liberating."

Walk Your Own Walk

Each religious tradition offers ritual, community, and
meaning that can help people feel better and find peace of
mind.

In fact, Dr. Hammerschlag's personal experience with
the native Americans has inspired him to become closer to
his own Jewish heritage. Now he draws from both traditions
for healing inspiration. "I sing my Jewish songs and I wear
my father's prayer shawl in the tepee," he adds.

"My Indian friends say that it does not matter in what language you sing; there are always at least two people who understand you—you and the Creator."

A Friend in Need

"Everybody needs somebody sometime," goes the old song. That's especially true for cancer patients. Research shows that emotional support from groups of people who are dealing with the same disease may do more than just improve the *quality* of life. It can *prolong* life as well.

"We were amazed to find that the women with terminal breast cancer who participated in support groups lived twice as long after joining the study, on the average, as women who were not assigned to a group," says David Spiegel, M.D., an associate professor of psychiatry and behavioral sciences at Stanford University. "What we expected to find was that women with metastatic breast cancer, half of whom die within two years, would have a better mental attitude and quality of life if they participated in support groups. We didn't expect to find greater life expectancy."

In their study, published in the British journal *Lancet,* Dr. Spiegel and his colleagues assigned 50 women with breast cancer that had spread to other parts of their bodies to weekly, 90-minute meetings in groups moderated by a psychiatrist and a social worker whose breast cancer was in remission. The groups were structured to allow the women to express their feelings about their illness and its impact on their lives. Group members encouraged their companions to be more assertive with their doctors, to learn how to draw strength from their ordeal and to help their families cope with it. The women were also instructed in self-hypnosis techniques to help them cope with pain as well. Another topic of discussion was the side effects of the aggressive cancer therapy they were all undergoing at that time. "The emphasis was on living with cancer. At no time did anyone raise the issue that this support might help people live longer," says Dr. Spiegel.

An additional 36 women who were being treated for spreading cancer, but who were not participating in support groups, were used as a random control group.

A Lease on Longer Life?

The support groups met regularly for a year, and the women were followed for 10 years. In 1988, when the study ended, all but three of the women had died, which was not surprising, since the average survival time for metastatic cancer is only 2 years after diagnosis. But the women who had been in the support groups had lived an average of 5 years following the discovery that their cancer had spread, while women without that experience had lived only an average of $3\frac{1}{2}$ years.

The fact that the three women who were still living ten years later were all in the support groups Dr. Spiegel terms "interesting" but not significant because of the small number. He doubts that they had remained in support groups for all that time.

"It seems that the crucial time for psychosocial support is when the person finds that their cancer has spread," he says. "It's when people find themselves 'walking that lonesome valley' toward death all by themselves. Cancer is a very isolating disease, and yet that very thing that isolates you is your ticket into a group that is experiencing the same tragedy."

There is strong evidence that social support can enhance survival in many diseases, not just cancer. Dr. Spiegel and his colleagues speculate that members of their groups may have been encouraged to cooperate more fully with their doctors, thus getting the maximum effect from their treatment. Group support appeared to relieve some of the depression that usually accompanies cancer, which also enabled the women to participate more fully in therapy. In addition, the hypnosis training may have aided in maintaining appetite and the willingness to exercise that prolonged survival.

"To me, the strength and significance of this therapy is that it's not a 'wish away your cancer' approach, but one that deals with the disease and the reality of death," says Dr. Spiegel. "I do not want anyone to interpret this study as implying that mental attitude can 'image' away cancer. What we found is that improving communication with doctors, controlling pain and other symptoms, and facing and mastering fears about death not only enhance the quality of life after a cancer diagnosis, but may help prolong life as well. I think such support groups should be routine in the care of all women with breast cancer."

Be Your Personal Best

Revitalize Your Love Life

You're frisky. He isn't. She has a headache. You don't. Or maybe you both have headaches—all the time. Or you both have jobs and kids to boot, so who has the energy to think about good sex? "Inhibited sexual desire" is what the experts call it. And New York City sex and marital therapist Shirley Zussman, Ed.D., says it's a concern for about 50 percent of the people who consult her. It can spring from many causes, "But I think the primary thing is fatigue and stress," says Dr. Zussman.

Whatever the cause, it takes an especially big toll on the sex lives of the over-30 crowd. Along with a few other common problems. Some emotional. Some physical. Some logistical—just finding time enough and space enough to be close.

But, contrary to naysayers everywhere, lack of sexual satisfaction in the middle years is not inevitable. After consulting experts across the country, *Prevention* found a whole array of cures for what ails sex after 30. The marital and sex therapists offered plenty of facts and techniques that can make for happier sex for a lifetime.

So for those interested parties who've declared better sex after 30 a lost cause, here are a few things to think about.

Get in Touch • "If there's one bit of advice I give to couples, especially those over 45, it's to look back and remember when they were dating," says marriage and sex therapist Judith Huffman Seifer, R.N., Ph.D., associate clinical pro-

242

fessor at the Wright State University School of Medicine, in Dayton, Ohio. "Intercourse was delayed, often until after marriage, and couples spent huge amounts of time touching—parking, necking, petting.

"I ask couples, 'How often do you pleasure one another in the way you used to, just touching, trailing your fingernails down his back, caressing the inside of her forearm?' Couples look at each other and giggle.

"That's why in sex therapy we say, no intercourse until we tell you otherwise, and work on touching instead. They get so turned on that we expect them to cheat! People rediscover one another, that the body doesn't work the same way it did. You practically have a whole new partner to deal with."

Take Time in Bed • Too many busy couples aim for what sex therapist Dagmar O'Connor calls "the 1-minute orgasm," meaning the fastest lovemaking possible. So they wind up feeling frustrated. O'Connor directs the sex-therapy program at St. Luke's-Roosevelt Hospital Center in New York and is the author of *How to Put the Love Back into Making Love*. She says, "I want to scream at these 1-minuters: 'Doesn't anyone remember when making love meant spending the whole day in bed?' "

Do an Emotional Housecleaning • "Built-up anger over the years is the biggest cause of lack of sexual desire," asserts Los Angeles therapist Barbara De Angelis, Ph.D. "When people think they have a sex problem, 90 percent of the time it has to do with little resentments, feelings of frustration about not being loved or acknowledged enough. Work on cleaning out whatever emotional clutter has built up between you. Those things kill passion."

Dating Can Still Get You to First Base • "If you don't have any fun together out of bed, it's pretty hard to have fun in bed," says Michael Castleman, author of *Sexual Solutions: A Guide for Men and the Women Who Love Them*. "People need to make time for nonsexual fun. Start dating again, go out to dinner, go to a play. Consciously put some of the spark back in the relationship. There's no guarantee that taking in plays and concerts will cause your partner to tear your clothes off," he adds, "but fun is fun, valuable for itself, and it helps people loosen up and relax. That's part of the key to enjoyable lovemaking."

You're Never Too Old for Safe Sex • Safe sex does much to ease your mind—not to mention reduce your risks. Besides, safe sex can be fun sex. The essence of safe sex is using condoms and avoiding high-risk partners. If you're uncertain about specifics, there are many excellent new books available to help steer women and men safely through the new, scarier sexual waters (see "Recommended Reading" on page 245).

Try a Tasteful "Cookbook" • If boredom is the problem, read up on new ideas, says sex counselor Robert O. Hawkins, Jr., Ph.D., professor of health sciences and associate dean at the State University of New York at Stony Brook. There are tasteful books that can be helpful. "I still recommend Alex Comfort's *Joy of Sex* and *More Joy of Sex*," he says. "They give people fresh ideas. But such books should be used the way they were intended, sort of like cookbooks, in which you select only the suggestions that suit you. I never used every recipe in the *Joy of Cooking*, and I don't know anyone who did. I select the recipes that appeal to me, and I don't consider it a hang-up that I don't want to cook up a chocolate, chili, and turkey dish called Turkey Mole."

Women, Enjoy Your Peak • It's true: Men reach their sexual peak (in terms of interest and responsiveness) in their teens, but women may not fully awaken to the joys of sex until their thirties or even forties. "We don't know why," says Virginia Sadock, M.D., director of the graduate education program in human sexuality at the New York University Medical Center. "There may be physical reasons: If a woman had children, she now has a greater blood flow to the genital area. Or it could be psychological: She may be more comfortable with her partner."

Laugh a Little • "Sex at its best is great play," asserts Steve Allen, Jr., M.D., a family practitioner, sexuality consultant, and humorist. Dr. Allen—who inherited his silliness from his famous dad—prescribes heavy doses of laughter for couples who are feeling tense in bed. "It doesn't mean you're not doing serious things," says Dr. Allen. "It means you're not taking yourself too seriously while doing them. Think of it as whimsy."

Try these whimsical strategies, he says: Arrive separately at a party and pick each other up, pretending you've just met. Play out your favorite movie or book love scene—how about the hilarious food scene from *Tom Jones,* in

---

Recommended Reading

Robert N. Butler, M.D., and Myrna I. Lewis. *Love & Sex after 60,* rev. ed. New York: Harper & Row, 1988.

Michael Castleman. *Sexual Solutions: A Guide for Men and the Women Who Love Them,* rev. ed. New York: Simon & Schuster, 1989. (Available from Self-Care Associates, P.O. Box 46–0066, San Francisco, CA 94146, $24.95 postage paid.)

Paula Brown Doress, Diana Laskin Siegal, and the Midlife and Older Women Book Project. *Ourselves, Growing Older.* New York: Simon & Schuster, 1987.

Dagmar O'Connor. *How to Put the Love Back into Making Love.* New York: Doubleday, 1989.

Paul Pearsall, Ph.D. *Super Marital Sex.* New York: Ballantine Books, 1987.

Philip Sarrel and Lorna Sarrel. *The Seven Stages of Adult Sexuality.* New York: Macmillan, 1984.

Beverly Whipple, Ph.D., R.N., and Gina Ogden, Ph.D. *Safe Encounters: How Women Can Say "Yes" to Pleasure and "No" to Unsafe Sex.* New York: McGraw-Hill, 1989.

which a (fully clothed) couple sensuously chomps their way through everything from melons to the inevitable bananas?

Changes in Men's Sexual Response May Be a Plus • By their thirties and forties, many men may need more direct stimulation of the penis to get an erection. They may not need to have a climax every time they make love. Erections may also be less firm, and the "recovery" time required between erections grows longer, says Dr. Sadock. "An 18-year-old man can climax up to eight times in 24 hours; when he's 35, once every 24 hours is more the norm," says Dr. Sadock. The good news: These changes can make men better lovers, says sexuality expert Paul A. Fleming, M.D., former editor of "Sex Over Forty" newsletter. "You may not be able to have sex three times in an hour, but you'll be better equipped to do it once and make it last an hour. So much for the myth of sexual decline!"

The "G-Spot" May Exist After All • If you're still looking for the infamous "G-spot" (said to be a sensitive spot on the front wall of the vagina), and enjoying the quest, you may have found it. In a recent article in *Medical Aspects of Human Sexuality,* David M. Quadagno, Ph.D., professor in medical sciences at Florida State University, reviews the controversial evidence as to whether the G-spot exists and comes to three safe-to-say conclusions: (1) Some (but not all) women do have a pressure-sensitive area on the front wall of the vagina, (2) some (but not all) women can have orgasms from strong rhythmic pressure inside the vagina without stimulation of the clitoris, and (3) fluid that some women produce at orgasm bears no similarity to male secretions, as G-spot enthusiasts believed.

Eat for Love • For men, there may be a good reason to watch their intake of saturated fats and cholesterol. These substances may lead to clogged blood vessels, reducing circulation. And reduced circulation in and around the penis is a common cause of impotence. So some experts speculate that in some men a high-fat diet may make erections more difficult to maintain, and that a low-fat diet could help avoid the problem.

Try It Three Times • "I always suggest to people that they try something new three times," says Dr. Hawkins. "The first time, you're concerned with, 'Am I doing it right, have I got my leg in the right position?' You may not like it just because it's new. By the second or third time, you may find it gives you a great deal of pleasure. But if by the third time you still don't like it, say, 'Let's look for something else.' "

There's No Such Thing as Normal Frequency • Sexual frequency, the number of times you make love in any given time, does tend to decline with age. "In the first 5 to 10 years, it's usually more than 2 times a week, but by 12 to 17 years of marriage, it's 1.4 times a week," says Dr. Seifer. But it's important to set your own standards, adds Castleman. "In fact, there are many very happily married people in their thirties, forties, and fifties who make love once every couple of weeks, once a month, and it's okay with both of them. People should consider what they really want, and not what they think they should want."

One, Two, Three, Do Your Kegels • Kegel exercises strengthen the pubococcygeus (PC) muscles, which stretch across the pelvic floor. Some women report stronger orgasms as a result of regular Kegels. Men can benefit from doing Kegels, too. Kegels give some men firmer erections, stronger orgasms, and more control over premature ejaculation. How to do a Kegel? First find the right muscles. They're the ones you use to stop your urine flow. Once you've located them, practice squeezing, holding for a few seconds and releasing. Half your contractions can be brief; hold the other half for 3 to 5 seconds. Start with 10 contractions a day, work up to 50 to 100 squeezes a day. They're silent—do them anywhere.

Get to Yes! • "Women especially need to learn to say, 'That feels good, keep doing that, ' " says Dr. Seifer. "The women's movement taught women to say no to what they don't want, but many women still don't know how to say yes to what they do want."

Exercise Improves Sex • Older men and women who exercise regularly have more sex, and enjoy it more, than nonactive people of the same age. "Exercise and physical activity permit most individuals to become at least 10 to 20 years younger physiologically than their chronological age," notes Raymond Harris, M.D., president of the Center for the Study of Aging, in Albany, New York. Recent evidence: Researchers at Bentley College in Waltham, Massachusetts, surveyed 160 people, age 40 to 80, all active in Masters swimming competition. They found that they had sex lives more like people in their late twenties or early thirties. Sexual encounters occurred 7.1 times a month for those in their forties, and 6.7 times a month for those 60 and older.

The Menopause Years Ain't What They Used to Be • And thank heavens! says Dr. Zussman. "Look around you at the women 45 to 55. This is a healthy population! They look young and terrific. Their children are out of the house; they're working, exercising, and studying. I think we're talking about a very different population than a decade ago. I'm an optimist; this period of life can be a new beginning." For most women, she says, menopause does not mean a decline in sexuality.

Sexual Activity Offers Women an Unexpected Benefit • Research indicates that, as long as older women have regular sex, they are likely to continue to lubricate normally and have a healthy vagina. In a New Jersey-Rutgers Medical School study, women 50 to 65 who had intercourse three or more times a month had no dryness problems.

The Best Is Yet to Be • Fact: Most people over 60 are very interested in sex. (Although it's perfectly okay to have little or no interest.) Fact: Most of them say the sex is as good as it was when they were younger. Fact: Most of them, male and female, say it's better than when they were younger. These are some of the findings of gerontological researchers Bernard Starr, Ph.D., and Marcella Weiner, Ed.D. Their data come from a survey of 800 seniors, ages 60 to 91.

Play the Question Game • "People who have a Hollywood approach to sex think, 'If he loved me, he would intuitively know what I want.' But he doesn't know, believe me. You have to talk about it," says Castleman. "That's why I came up with the Question Game."

Here's how it works: You and your partner separately write down everything you want the other person to do for you affectionwise. "Be completely selfish and be specific," says Castleman. "Don't write 'I want him to be more sensitive.' Write 'I want him to give me a hug and kiss when I come home from work.' And a man cannot write 'I want her to be sexier.' He should write 'I wish she would wear lace silk pajamas.' "

Then rank the list. At the top, put the things that are easiest for you to ask for, working down to those that are the most difficult. Don't show the list to your partner yet. Sit down with a calendar and make a set of dates with each other—once every month or two. Beginning on the first date, you and your partner tell each other the request at the top of each of your lists. "No one is under any obligation to grant the other person's request. Your only commitment is to listen carefully and not dismiss the request out-of-hand," says Castleman.

"The first thing that happens," he says, "is most people only come up with six to eight requests. That in itself is a revelation; they realize they're close to the relationship they want. And then the first requests almost invariably have to do with things that don't take place in bed. The number one request when I was doing this counseling, from both men and women, was for more cuddling when watching TV.

"Then six months down the road, you get to the more difficult requests. By then you've had practice talking about sex, and the person who is being asked to do something has already granted a half-dozen requests and can more honestly say, 'I can't do that.' So the asker may be annoyed, but also thinks, 'Well, my partner granted most of my requests; this relationship is pretty good!' "

You Can Counteract Dryness • In menopause, intercourse can sometimes be more uncomfortable because the vaginal tissue can become dry and thin. But lubricants can usually resolve the problem. In more troublesome cases, a gynecologist can prescribe vaginal estrogen cream, or a woman might want to consider hormone-replacement therapy. Talk to your gynecologist, says Dr. Zussman. "You don't need to be uncomfortable."

Beware of Dennis the Menace • With more women in their thirties having children, older couples are discovering the Dennis-the-Menace syndrome. That's the term New Haven sex counselors Lorna Sarrel and Philip Sarrel, M.D., use to describe the dampening effect that children can have on a couple's sex life.

But experts say that the degree of "menace" changes with the children's age. They offer these age-specific tips.

• Infants can be especially tough on your sex life, at least at first. Women who have just delivered are understandably less likely to feel amorous. "They're tired, they're nursing, they're juggling their husband's and baby's demand for intimacy," says Sandra Leiblum, Ph.D., professor of clinical psychiatry at the University of Medicine and Dentistry of New Jersey, Robert Wood Johnson Medical School. She counsels patience. "Men get frustrated. But the situation really can change as the marriage develops."
• Sending toddlers or children off to day care and elementary school can bring on a second honeymoon, says Dr. Leiblum.
• "The teenager with the blaring music and unpredictable hours can get in the way again," says Dr. Sadock. Get a good bedroom lock, splurge on weekend vacations as often

as you can afford them, she advises. "Usually it's better if you get out of the house because you never know when an adolescent will walk back in."

The good news: The Sarrels say that although the Dennis-the-Menace syndrome is the rule, there are many exceptions. "One couple described the excitement of 'hiding' from the kids the way they used to hide from parents when they were 18."

Get Counseling • Need more help? Talk to a physician if there are medical concerns. Marriage or sex counselors can listen to your problems and make suggestions. Sex therapy is a process in which a couple meet regularly to talk with a sex therapist, who often tells them to go home and do progressive exercises in touching and communication.

For a national directory of certified, qualified sex counselors and therapists, send $10 to the American Association of Sex Educators, Counselors and Therapists (AASECT), 435 N. Michigan Ave., Suite 1717, Chicago, IL 60611. Your family physician, local medical center, or county medical society can refer you to appropriate professionals.

Older Sex Is Slow and Sensuous • "People can have sex, and love it, well into old age. But they must keep in mind that where they used to get excited in 10 seconds, it will take longer to get an erection or lubricate," notes Dr. Sadock. Older people who don't know that more time and more direct stimulation are needed may give up too soon, making problems worse. Once you understand the difference that age has made, you can have the time of your life!

A 72-year-old woman told Dr. Starr and Dr. Weiner, "Our sex is so much more relaxed, I know my body better, and we know each other better—sex is unhurried and the best in our lives."

Erection Problems May Not Be All in Your Mind • Contrary to popular belief, an inability to get an erection need not be due to emotional difficulties. Several studies have shown that many cases have physical causes, like high blood pressure, artery disease, pelvic-nerve disorders, and diabetes. (The telling clue is whether the man has erections not associated with sex, like in the morning. If so, the problem is unlikely to be physical.) Medical care and lifestyle improvements can change things.

Medications Can Cause Impotence • Some prescription drugs, including cimetidine (Tagamet), blood pressure medicines, and antidepressants can bring on temporary impotence. "Sometimes it takes some careful detective work to pinpoint the offending medication, but it is often possible to make substitutions," says Albert McBride, M.D., national spokesperson for the Impotence Foundation in Los Angeles, California.

Be Good to Yourself • Every sex therapist consulted agreed that women or men who are alone, and who miss sensuality, may benefit from the release of providing it for themselves.

"Give yourself a special evening as if you had a special lover," says O'Connor. "Buy yourself a bouquet of flowers, pick up some nice books to get your mind flowing, romantic novels or whatever you like, play your favorite music. Relax and stroke your body. Giving yourself this kind of attention is very good for you," says O'Connor. Through self-stimulation, women can promote vaginal health, which can mean less pain during intercourse if they do become sexually involved again.

It's Never Too Late • Some women who never experienced orgasm when they were younger often do much later because they simply make the effort. A few women even become orgasmic for the first time in their senior years. "My favorite lady was a 73-year-old widow. She came to me and told me that she wanted to have one orgasm before she died," recalls O'Connor. "Well, now she's multiorgasmic, has a new boyfriend, and is living in Florida!"

Take the Workaholic Test • In the after-30 era, one of the biggest obstacles to satisfying sex is overwork. Dr. Zussman says that a clue that too much work is what's cramping your love style is this: Once you start making love, you enjoy it, but it's getting to it that's difficult.

Check for Boredom • "The most common issue I find with midlife couples is sexual boredom," says Dr. Seifer. "Couples get tired of doing the same thing, in the same way, in the same place."

How do you know if boredom is the problem? Ask yourself this question, says Dr. Seifer: "When you go on vacation and find yourself in a new place like a hotel, do you find that your sexual relationship gets more exciting— then seems to fall back into a rut when you get back home?"

Avoid the Middle-Years' Slipup • Women need to remember that it may be possible for them to become pregnant even in the early stages of menopause. Even if it's been a few months since they had a menstrual period, it may not be their last. Experts recommend using birth control for a year after the last period because hormones are still settling down, and another period can follow what seemed to be the last one.

Instant Recall

By Andrew Roblin

After my wife and I moved into our home, a neighbor came over with a gift: a tissue-box cover embroidered with an *R*, the initial of our surname. "How thoughtful of you . . ." I groped for my neighbor's name. She had introduced herself a week before. ". . . Mrs. Farmer."

"I'm not Mrs. Farmer." Mrs. Farmer was a different neighbor. "I'm Emily."

I'm not alone in forgetting names. From time to time, most of us find ourselves on the losing end of the name game. If only we had perfect memories, like computers do. Good news: With a few easy strategies, most of us can rival—even exceed—the computer's prowess.

Meeting Mrs. What's-Her-Name

Exceed? Yes. In a sense, our memories are already better than computers': We can recognize faces in an instant and, often, match them with the right names. Computers can't. Not yet, anyway. Recognizing a face prompts us to consult a mental file containing all we know about the person, says Michael L. Epstein, Ph.D., chairman of the Psychology Department at Rider College, Lawrenceville, New Jersey. Flipping through the file should turn up the right name. Sometimes, though, the name eludes us.

Often, that's because we haven't concentrated on learning the name when we first heard it (see "Beat These Memory Busters" on page 255 for other things that can disrupt memory). When I met Emily, for instance, I concentrated on making a good impression, not on her name.

Step one to better memory: When you first meet, concentrate on the person and her name.

Step two: Care enough to use the mnemonic devices, the memory aids, that follow.

Okay. You're concentrating. You care. Now step three: Choose an appropriate mnemonic device. Perhaps you can take your cue from the person's features. My new acquaintance's hairline looks like an *M*. Phonetically, *em* stands for Emily.

Rhyming is another name saver: Jill's on the Pill. Frank broke the bank. Gail's like a whale. If you can rhyme a name, you can embed it in your memory.

If no rhyme comes to mind, use the person's name to invent an unforgetable image. Harris is an easy name to remember this way. Imagine Harris with grossly exaggerated hair: a sky-high bouffant or a pompadour the size of a tidal wave.

For a name like Yastrzemski, try another tack. Imagine

Beat These Memory Busters

Stress. Memory failures seem to happen most when we're out of our usual routine, tired, or under stress. Pressure to remember adds to stress. Stress can preoccupy us, diverting our attention from what we try to remember. And all this makes us less likely to remember names.

Anxiety. Anxiety, worries, and obsessions reduce attention span. Reduced attention reduces memory.

Depression. Problems concentrating and remembering are sometimes symptoms of depression. "We don't know exactly how depression interferes with memory," says Norman Foster, M.D., director of the cognitive disorders program, University of Michigan Medical School, Ann Arbor. "But depression does affect brain chemistry, including three chemicals that appear related to memory: dopamine, noradrenaline and acetylcholine."

Treatment of depression often reduces memory problems in depressed people.

Medications. Sleeping medications, sedatives, and tranquilizers can interfere with memory by reducing alertness and attention. Remember, though, memory loss may be less significant than the diseases these drugs treat. Consult your doctor before changing medications.

Illnesses. Memory loss can accompany Alzheimer's, Parkinson's, and Lyme disease; alcoholism; and thyroid, thiamine, and vitamin B_{12} deficiency.

Age. As we grow older, our powers of concentration tend to decline. That doesn't mean we have to spend the rest of our lives asking acquaintances to repeat their names. With mnemonic techniques and daily mental stimulation, we can actually improve memory as we age.

your neighbor doing something that sounds like Yastrzem-ski: You strum a ski. True, it's a silly image—silly enough to be memorable.

Or perhaps you know of a celebrity with the same name. If you follow baseball, you might imagine your neighbor hitting the way the great batter Carl Yastrzemski did.

You can use imagery to associate your neighbor's name with what it means. If the name is Farmer, picture her driving a combine through a field full of wheat. The name is Smith? Picture a blacksmith over a forge.

Use these techniques any way that works for you. The only limitation is your imagination. "The last syllable of my name is 'stein,' " says Dr. Epstein. "To remember it, think of drinking beer out of a stein.

"A prominent feature on my face happens to be my nose. It might be the first thing you notice about me. Instead of a nose on my face, picture a stein. Better yet, turn it upside down. Then you've got 'up stein,' which is close to Epstein."

Encountering a Roomful of Names

Remembering the names of a group of people requires the same steps: concentrate, care, and choose a mnemonic device.

But remembering more names is more challenging. Our short-term memory holds an average of only five new names, plus or minus two. So the trick is to get the names quickly into long-term memory, which has infinite storage capacity.

Before you can transfer the names to long-term memory, though, you have to get them well into short-term memory. When meeting several people, one of the best ways is with a device you can remember by its acronym, SALT.

Say each person's name as you meet them. "Nice to meet you, Mr. Smith." Often, when we're introduced to people, we don't get their names because we're thinking of ourselves. Saying the name forces you to process it. While you're at it, look for a cue in the person's face, in the meaning or sound of the name, that you can use as a mnemonic.

Ask questions. For instance, "Is that S-M-I-T-H or S-M-Y-T-H-E?" You may know the spelling, but asking about it makes you concentrate on the name. And, when you ask questions, you get information about the person—information that may offer great cues to help remember the name.

Learn by repetition. Say the name again. "Nice day for a party, Mr. Smith."

Terminate the conversation with the name. "It was a pleasure meeting you, Mr. Smith." You've now said the name at least four times. And the last thing you've said is Mr. Smith's name.

All this takes time. You'll have to spend a minute or two talking to each person. You need time to learn names.

After you've salted away about three names, take a moment to mentally repeat them. Look again at each person you've met and rehearse their names. When you're comfortable with those, you're ready to learn three more.

An hour later, review the names you want to keep in long-term memory and visualize the persons (including how they walk and move) that go with them, says Irene B. Colsky, Ed.D., an adjunct professor at the University of Miami, who leads memory-building seminars. Ask yourself, "Who did I meet this morning?" Repeat the reviewing process several times over the next 24 hours. Without review, you'll lose 50 percent of what you learned.

Of course, there's nothing wrong with writing everyone's name. Normally, though, few bring pad and pencil to a party. If you use mnemonic devices, you won't need to.

Recalling a Face—But Not the Name

Recognizing a face is easier than recalling the name that goes with it. It's like the difference between answering a multiple-choice and an essay question. When we see a face, or the answer to a multiple-choice question, all we have to do is recognize that it's familiar. When we try to recall someone's name, or answer an essay question, we have to dredge the information from our memories. Tension, especially self-induced pressure to come up with a name, makes that job harder. "Imagine the information is sitting somewhat precariously on a loading platform," says Dr. Colsky. "The harder you try to reach the information, the more difficult it is to recall it. If you're not careful, you can push it right off the platform, and then you have difficulty getting it back again. So what you want to do is push the information onto the platform and make it more secure. But you can't do that with tension and anxiety."

The solution? Relax; take a deep breath. Then ignore the name for the moment. Think instead of the person—her most prominent features, the things she has told you about herself, the places you've seen her, anything that might prompt her name to surface. "I call it the hole-in-the-doughnut technique," says Dr. Colsky. "You get pieces of information all around the hole. And before you know it, you've got the whole doughnut. Then the name pops into your mind.

"Have you ever found when you're not thinking of a name it comes right to mind? That's because you've removed the stress and anxiety that cause the block. So stall and relax. Talk about the weather, anything. Before you know it, you're using her name, because you're not concentrating on it."

If that doesn't help, try going through the alphabet. Does the name begin with *A, B, C* or *D*? A letter may give you a hook that will fish the name to the surface, even if it's in an unexpected way. The letter *E* may not bring Emily to mind, for instance, but *M* might.

And if you still draw a blank? Don't be ashamed to say, "I'm sorry. Your name is on the tip of my tongue, but I can't call it to mind. Would you please repeat your name?" People will be flattered to know you care about their names.

Find Some Joy
in Every Day

Ah, happiness. Is it truly elusive? Or is it just our unrealistic goals and expectations that keep pushing it out of reach?

Social psychologist Ed Diener, Ph.D., of the University of Illinois, votes for the latter. In ongoing research into expectations and goals, Diener has found that impossibly high goals can destroy any hope of experiencing day-to-day delights. And consistently experiencing day-to-day joys, he says, not the occasional highs, "are the key to predicting happiness."

Diener, along with psychologists Richard H. Smith, Ph.D., and Douglas Wedell, Ph.D, reported in a recent study published by the *Journal of Personality and Social Psychology* that the quality of people's expectations makes a big difference in their level of happiness.

The researchers asked 158 college students with high expectations of themselves to evaluate how they'd feel if, for example, they failed a test or received low wages. What they learned was that the participants felt that having their expectations lowered by these small failures was actually helpful. They made the students more realistic about their life plans and happier with daily progress toward their goals.

It's the age-old message about life being a journey rather than a destination, explains Dr. Diener. "People in our culture are encouraged to have high expectations," he says. And those high expectations can be damaging in one of two ways—either people experience disappointment when life doesn't meet those lofty goals, or people become disillusioned because they live only for a peak experience and everyday life can't match up all of the time.

Balancing Highs and Lows

Dr. Diener uses the example of a honeymoon. "If you can enjoy people around you and enjoy the activities you are doing, then when highs come along occasionally, like

259

going on your honeymoon or winning an award, they're fine and they add a little bit to your happiness, but that's not really what happiness is. Happiness is a long-term thing." People may live for the honeymoon and expect their entire married life to be like that when it in fact is made up of all kinds of experiences.

It's not that you shouldn't go on honeymoons or long pleasure-filled vacations, but you should take stock of how you perceive these kinds of experiences. "If you enjoy the day-to-day things that you are doing, then you're all right," Dr. Diener says. If you only live for those planned-for and rarely lived highs, then chances are your everyday life may be full of lows.

Financial budgeting offers an even more mundane explanation of the problem. In their paper, the researchers cite an earlier study about the ways in which people allot their salary from week to week. What they found is that those people who let themselves spend a little more than average most days and then enforce a few lean days were much happier than those folks who were scrimping every minute to have a spending blitz at the end of the month.

Dr. Diener also is not suggesting that you refrain from difficult, long-term goals (like amassing a savings account), but he does recommend that you focus on the short-term goals and the activities that lead to such big accomplishments. "Be a little bit happy most of the time," Dr. Diener advises. "If you want to be president, you better not worry too much about actually being president, but you'd better enjoy the everyday activities that it takes—like being in politics."

Reverse Dementia
with Aspirin

Dementia. Mental deterioration. Literally losing your mind. It's something we all fear, sometimes even more than the loss of something more physical. After all, our mind is what we truly are. It's "us."

But dementia is not entirely separate from the more physical world of, say, our heart or our blood vessels. In fact, it's long been suspected that the same reduced blood flow of atherosclerosis that threatens our heart health might also cause one form of dementia ("multi-infarct," the second most common type after Alzheimer's) by starving the brain of blood-borne oxygen.

One study involving thousands of physicians provided strong evidence that an aspirin a day has the potential to protect our heart from such circulatory problems.

Now, a startling new study has shown that the same aspirin a day can actually lessen the effects of dementia related to poor circulation in the elderly.

That's right—we're not talking prevention here. We're talking improvement. We're talking about *less* confusion, *less* dependency on others, and a higher quality of life—all *after* dementia has reared its ugly head. *And* a longer life to boot.

70 People Tell the Tale

Researchers from the University of Houston and Baylor College of Medicine working in the Cerebral Blood Flow Laboratory of the Veterans Affairs Medical Center began by selecting 70 people (average age 67) who were already suffering some level of (non-Alzheimer's) dementia.

They were broken into two groups. In one, 37 people received a single 325-milligram aspirin tablet a day. The 33 members of the other group, matched for age, sex, medical status, and level of dementia, received exactly the same kinds of treatments and therapies—except that they took no aspirin.

The results of the three-year study, as reported in the June 1989 issue of the *Journal of the American Geriatric Society,* are nothing short of remarkable.

When the study began, everyone took a test called the Cognitive Capacity Screening Exam (CCSE) that evaluates your mental state at the time you take it. In someone with progressive dementia, you expect to see lower scores over the years.

But for the people who took aspirin, those scores went *up* instead of down. At the end of the first year, the average score was 17.2 percent higher. At the end of two years it was 21.4 percent higher.

Putting it simply, these people had improved their mental capacity by more than one-fifth. They had regained a lot of the working thought processes that dementia had previously taken away.

The scores of the people who didn't get the aspirin declined. At the end of a year those scores were 5.3 percent lower. The people were getting worse—more confused, more dependent on others.

As the study points out, the difference between the two groups wasn't limited to test scores.

"The aspirin-treated patients also showed improvement in their activities of daily living and became less dependent upon others, which was not seen among the control [non-aspirin-taking] patients," the researchers report.

And Fewer Strokes, Too!

Aspirin did more than just help these lucky people think more clearly. Those who took aspirin had half the number of transient ischemic attacks (TIAs, or ministrokes) as those who went without.

In the group that didn't get the aspirin there were eight full-blown strokes. In the aspirin group there were two.

There were eight deaths overall: five in the group that didn't get aspirin compared to only three in the aspirin group.

But *Only* One a Day!

It seems that *one* aspirin a day is very effective at opening clogged blood vessels (possibly by dissolving tiny little clots) and thus allowing more oxygen-rich blood to reach the gray matter areas of the brain.

In fact, measurements showed an increase in cerebral blood flow (CBF) to these essential areas in those who took aspirin.

However, this is a case where one may be great, but two is too many. The researchers warn that increasing the dose to just *two* aspirin (650 milligrams) or the equivalent in other aspirin-like drugs (such as nonsteroidal anti-inflammatory drugs like ibuprofen and other drugs often used to treat arthritis) *reverses* the effect.

Too much aspirin, or other aspirin-like drugs, they say, *reduces* CBF and may worsen dementia.

So don't take two in the hopes that you'll think more clearly twice as fast.

Body-Care Updates

Soft Touch: Do's and Don'ts for Beautiful Hands

Few things are more feminine than lovely hands. While you can't do anything about the size and shape of your hands, you can control their overall condition and appearance. Even short fingers look elegant if the skin is soft, the cuticles smooth, and the nails manicured. *Prevention* asked Lia Schorr, New York City skin-care expert, to share her favorite hand-care hints.

DO give your hands the same gentle cleansing you give your face. Use a mild liquid cleanser or a nonsoap cleansing bar to wash your hands.

DON'T rub your hands dry after washing. Instead, pat dry and apply moisturizing cream.

DO use a moisturizing lotion or cream that contains sunscreen. Constant sunscreen use helps fade brown age spots and delays the start of new ones. If your hand lotion doesn't come in a sunscreen formula, use sunscreen under your lotion. Apply it 20 minutes before you go out. Try the convenient new sunscreen towelettes. They fit handily into a purse or backpack.

DO help fade age spots by using a bleaching cream containing hydroquinone. Always use a sunscreen over a bleaching cream; sun exposure undoes the good work done by the cream. And be patient: You'll probably have to wait several months to see results.

DON'T skip your cuticles and the base of your nails when you massage moisturizing lotion or cream into your fingers. This extra attention can pay off with more supple skin that's less prone to hangnails.

DO wear cotton-lined rubber gloves when doing household chores. The chemicals in common cleaners can dry and irritate your skin.

DON'T leave your rubber gloves on for too long. If you already have a problem with dermatitis, make it no longer than 10 minutes at a time. Rubber doesn't breathe, so perspiration is locked in, causing further irritation.

DO push cuticles back lightly, with your towel, after your bath or shower. They're hydrated then, so they're more pliable and less likely to crack.

DO give your hands a special heat treatment after a shower. For softening, pat them almost dry, apply hand cream, and cover completely with plastic wrap or gloves for at least an hour. This helps retain heat and trap moisture for deeper penetration.

DO apply a rich hand cream at bedtime. The cream can soak into your skin instead of rubbing off during the day as you do your many tasks. Give dry hands a treat by applying petroleum jelly to damp hands and covering them with white cotton gloves while you sleep.

DO a thorough but gentle job on calluses with a two-step beauty regimen of sloughing and moisturizing. At your nightly bath, gently rub a pumice stone over the callused area. Massage gently for a few minutes. Then apply a heavy cream or petroleum jelly.

DO use only nonacetone nail-polish remover. It's less drying to your nails and less irritating to the skin around them.

DO relaxing exercises to keep hands limber, improve circulation, and fight fatigue:

• Raise your hands over your head. Inhale deeply and count to five, then exhale slowly while lowering your hands to your sides. Next, shake both hands vigorously while holding loosely from the wrists. Repeat five times.
• Place one hand in your lap, palm upward. Use the opposite fist to massage the inside of the palm in a circular motion. Switch hands and repeat.

• Smooth on hand cream and massage it into each finger separately, working in circular motions from the base of the finger to the tip. Then work the cream into the back and palm of your hand.

DO treat yourself monthly to a full, professional manicure. It can give you a good pattern to follow for well-groomed hands and nails. As you establish your own routine, a professional manicure can provide maintenance in those areas that are difficult to do yourself.

Tips to Tackle the Hidden Causes of Bad Breath

Pssst! About your . . . uh . . . well . . . your breath. I didn't want to say anything but . . . as a friend I just wanted to tell you: Bad breath—a rampant STD (Socially Terrifying Disease)—can happen to you for the strangest, most unexpected reasons.

The not-so-strange reasons you can handle. If you eat the wrong food, you try a breath mint, brush/floss/rinse, or hide out until you're presentable to the public. If you have gum disease (which can be very mild, causing only minor gum bleeding), you're dealing with the most common cause of bad breath. The answer is usually just basic oral hygiene.

But some little-known instigators of bad breath are trickier. And they have a way of doing their worst just as you're walking into the most important meeting of your entire life.

So in the interests of socially acceptable breath the world over, here is a rogues' gallery of offbeat breath spoilers, with strategies for clearing the air once and for all.

Drugs • Antihistamines, decongestants, antianxiety drugs, diuretics—any drug that dries your mouth—can create a perfect environment for bad-breath bacteria. Saliva is slightly acidic and normally suppresses bacteria. But when saliva dries up, bacteria reproduce like a band of bunnies.

If you're taking mouth-drying medication only temporarily, frequent sips of water can overcome the dryness problem. If you're taking mouth-drying drugs for a longer time, your doctor or dentist may suggest you try artificial saliva. It duplicates the wetting properties of natural saliva.

But check with your doctor before discontinuing any prescription medication. Bad breath is probably less of an evil than the problem the drug controls.

Stress • Stress may reduce the flow of saliva, producing mouth dryness and giving odor-causing bacteria a chance to embarrass you. That's why stress and bad breath may make for a vicious circle. If someone has bad breath and becomes stressed about it, the stress may further dry the mouth and worsen bad breath.

Giving a speech, for instance, may start the cycle. If you're nervous, the stress may reduce your salivary flow. And talking may further dry you out. So if you're making a speech or preparing for some other stressful situation and are concerned about your breath, it may be a good idea to drink plenty of water and suck on a sugarless breath mint beforehand.

Mouth Sores • Cankers, bites, and other mouth sores can make breath bad in two ways. First, in extreme cases, the sore itself may cause an odor. Second, and much more common, the sore discourages thorough tooth cleaning. It hurts, so to avoid the hurt, we sometimes skip brushing and flossing nearby teeth, leaving food particles lying about. Mouth bacteria then feast on the particles, excreting sulfurous gases that make breath bad.

To stop the hurt and make brushing a breeze, apply an anesthetic gel that can provide a protective coating. It numbs the sore, letting you clean your teeth without irritation. Even with an anesthetic coating in place, try not to disturb the sore. The longer it takes to heal, the longer brushing can be a pain.

To speed healing, rinse your mouth with 1 teaspoon of salt in 1 cup of warm water. The salt solution cleans mouth tissue, stimulating it to heal. Don't use a mouthwash made with alcohol, which irritates and dries sores.

One other commonsense tip: While the sore is healing, eat bland, soft foods. Avoid nuts, which can abrade the sore, and irritating, acidic fruit.

"Desert Mouth" • If you do a lot of extra gaping and yakking—two open-mouthed pastimes beloved of many—you can instigate bad breath. They can dry out the mouth, leaving bad-breath bacteria to their own devices. And most of us tend to sleep open-mouthed—a cause of dreaded "morning breath," or "swamp mouth."

Rinsing with or sipping water helps restore a dry mouth to a pristine state. So does eating certain foods (because eating stimulates saliva production), followed by brushing and flossing. The right foods are those that don't add to the problem (as garlic or onions might). Even better are cleansing foods, such as celery and carrots—fibrous, mouthscrubbing foods that tend not to stick to teeth.

Hormones • For years, doctors have reported that women tend to complain of bad breath during menstruation. And years ago a scientific study suggested a reason for menstrual bad breath (*Journal of International Medical Research*). Lower progesterone and estrogen levels during menstruation may trigger increased shedding of cells from the mouth's mucous membranes, says the study's chief author, Joseph Tonzetich, Ph.D., professor of oral biology at the University of British Columbia, Vancouver. The cells provide extra food for mouth bacteria, increasing their numbers and their production of bad-breath gases.

Ovulation, too, may contribute to bad breath. High levels of estrogen and other sex hormones at ovulation apparently prompt a rise in the natural fluid that comes from the notch where teeth and gums meet. The fluid is rich in leukocytes (white blood cells) and other blood components. "These factors and fluid provide food for mouth bacteria," says Dr. Tonzetich. "They also act as cofactors, meaning they help the bacteria grow." The result can be an increase in the intensity of bad breath, particularly in women with gum disease, which also seems to worsen with high estrogen. Fortunately, this bad-breath peak lasts only a day or so.

Also fortunately, curing "hormonal" breath doesn't require extra effort, just normal effort: Basic dental hygiene can do the trick (see "Getting a Breath of Fresh Air" on page 270).

Preparing an Italian Dinner • Believe it or not, handling lots of garlic, as a chef might, can cause garlic breath. An often-cited experiment found that garlic rubbed into the feet of a 12-year-old boy later tainted his breath. Aromatic substances in garlic seem to enter through the pores, arrive in the bloodstream, get released in the lungs, and are then exhaled.

When you eat garlic, by the way, its aromatic components still follow a strange bloodstream-to-lungs route, which is why you can't always dampen the odor by simply brushing or rinsing. The same is true for other aromatic foods, such as onions, curry, and alcohol. Not only that, but the aromatic factors of all these foods can come out through pores when you sweat.

Until the aromatic substances dissipate, about 24 hours after they enter the bloodstream, the best approach to this type of bad breath is masking. You just overwhelm the odor with something pleasant. Parsley, peppermint, and wintergreen follow the same metabolic route as garlic, releasing pleasant aromatic substances through the lungs. It's okay to chew raw parsley, but get your peppermint and wintergreen in chewing gums and breath mints.

And here's a preemptive solution: cooking. Heat breaks down the aromatics in garlic and onions, making them much less offensive.

Sinusitis • Like mouth sores, sinus infections can cause bad breath two ways. First, a stuffy nose promotes mouth

Getting a Breath of Fresh Air

To eliminate the most common causes of bad breath:

• Every day, brush twice and floss once. Brushing and flossing disrupt the bacteria that cause gum disease, the chief cause of bad breath.
• "Gum disease" may call to mind a decayed, festering jaw. But it starts innocuously, with gums becoming inflamed and bleeding easily. In time, though, inflammation can lead to infected pockets between teeth and gums, even tooth loss. Whatever its stage, gum disease involves bacteria, damaged tissue, and, often, powerfully sour breath.
• Mild gum disease clears up with two or three days of brushing and flossing. More advanced cases may take a few weeks.
• Brush your tongue. The tongue's hairlike cells collect fetid mouth bacteria. To scrub away the bacteria, dentists recommend brushing the tongue at least once or twice a week.
• Brush the walls of the mouth, too. Doing so helps remove damaged cells before bacteria start feasting on them. Use a brush with soft, rounded bristles to avoid injuring your mouth.
• Use mouthwash. Provided you don't have a mouth sore or a wound from dental surgery, rinsing with mouthwash can help, too. Any mouthwash masks bad breath, overwhelming it with flavoring. But this masking is temporary, lasting only an hour or so.
• You'll get longer-lasting results—up to 3 hours—from mouthwash that reduces the buildup of bad-breath bacteria. The active ingredients to look for are thymol, eucalyptol, methyl salicylate, and menthol. In prescription mouthwashes, the key breath-cleansing factor is chlorhexidine.
• If bad breath persists, see a dentist or doctor. Unrelenting bad breath may signify serious dental and other problems: food impacted in a cavity, ulcers, diabetes, even kidney or liver failure.

breathing, drying up saliva and allowing bacteria to flourish. Drinking fluids, as we said, can counterattack.

Second, there's postnasal drip. In severe cases, bad-smelling fluid drips from the sinuses, imparting an unpleasant odor to the breath. If you have this kind of bad breath, see a doctor. You'll probably need antibiotics to clear up the infection.

Until the antibiotics kick in, try irrigating your nose with a few squirts of saline solution (in the ratio of $\frac{1}{2}$ teaspoon of salt to 1 cup of water). The salt water washes away the buildup of secretions and bacteria in the nasal cavity, helping to resolve the underlying infection.

High-Fat Diets • Some researchers suspect that diets high in fatty meats and cheeses, butter, and whole milk may cause bad breath. The theory is that, as garlic does, certain fats may contain smelly aromatic substances that we metabolize and exhale. Possible solution: If other causes of bad breath have been eliminated, try cutting back on fatty foods in your diet and replacing them with carbohydrates, such as vegetables, fruits, and whole grains.

Tonsilloliths • Repeated tonsillitis, the well-known infection of the tonsils, sets the stage for bad breath in an odd, unexpected way. You see, tonsils are covered with tiny craters. With chronic tonsillitis, some tissue may die, eventually turning into a soft substance that plugs the craters. These plugs catch small bits of calcium from food and saliva, turning into hard, white particles called tonsilloliths. Tonsilloliths can be the source of mouth odor. They may produce coughing, gagging, and the feeling that something bad tasting and foreign is in the mouth. One doctor reports that they occur in as many as 10 percent of his patients. Curing this kind of bad breath is usually simple. Poking the tonsil with a finger often expels the tonsillolith.

"If you can't dislodge a tonsillolith yourself, see your physician. He or she may be able to remove it painlessly. But if the problem persists, your doctor may recommend a tonsillectomy," says Fred G. Fedok, M.D., assistant professor of otolaryngology, head and neck surgery at the Hershey Medical Center in Pennsylvania.

Bridgework • Bridges are a particular challenge to clean, since a thin film of food residue can stick to the metal clasp that sits against the tooth. To clean the clasp, use a special clasp brush (it looks like a miniature Christmas tree).

Bridge wearers also have to watch for the accumulation of food, dead cells, and bacteria on the living gum underneath the artificial tooth. Using floss or a special plastic device that looks like a needle can clean away this buildup.

Dental Work • Just as a mouth sore can set off bad-breath alarms, so can wounds following dental surgery. During surgery, cells die and some bleeding occurs. Mouth bacteria chow down and, as an after-dinner trick, stink up your mouth.

Dental surgery leads to bad breath another way, too. A wisdom-tooth extraction, for instance, leaves a socket where food and bacteria may lodge.

But it's difficult—and risky—to clean the socket with a toothbrush or toothpick; you may cram debris into the socket and cause infection. Instead, clean the socket by rinsing your mouth with the salt solution mentioned on page 268. But rinse gently: You don't want to wash away scar tissue before the socket heals.

If bad breath persists while any dental wound is healing, mask the odor with sugarless breath mints.

Bounce Back from Back Pain

You stoop over to pick up the morning paper. You twist around to grab your seat belt. You reach up to the top shelf for a can of paint.

And you feel a twinge.

Lower back pain: one of the most common maladies

that makes mankind miserable. Four out of five people will fall victim to the twinge during their lifetime. That makes back pain the second most frequent cause of work loss in people under the age of 45 (behind only the common cold).

Fortunately, many physicians are now changing the way they treat common lower back pain. And that's good, because a lot of "older" cures were as likely to aggravate the problem as solve it.

Today's more enlightened practitioner realizes that the key to bouncing back from a bad back is a little common sense and a program of preventive maintenance, says Mark D. Brown, M.D., Ph.D., professor and chairman of the Department of Orthopaedics and Rehabilitation at the University of Miami School of Medicine.

In fact, he feels that the great majority of potential future back pain sufferers could probably sidestep the doctor's office altogether if they'd get up now and do the same thing that he would advise them to do after their back had actually gone bad: exercise.

A workout that strengthens the lower back and abdominal muscles is the perfect before *or* after the fact prescription, he says. It can prevent back pain. It can help people who are presently in pain. And it can help prevent that pain from coming back after it's gone.

A Fit Back Is Hard to Hurt

"If you have a propensity for back pain—and 60 percent of us who are over the age of 30 do—proper exercise will mean less frequent and less severe attacks," says Dr. Brown. "Even if you *do* have an attack, the fact that you have been exercising means you'll get over it quicker."

As an example, he points to Joe Montana, the superstar quarterback of the San Francisco 49ers. Many thought he might never play the game again after he underwent surgery for a herniated disk.

"He not only came back but was able to play the way he had before he was injured," notes Dr. Brown. "He's a great example of how a person with a back injury can resume full activity because he was in good shape to begin with and was highly motivated to maintain an intensive conditioning program."

Scientific studies also support the value of proper exercise.

Prevention Is Possible

Dr. Brown explains that one study that examined firefighters especially demonstrates how personal fitness can *prevent* back injuries.

"The men's fitness levels were evaluated, and they were divided into two groups; one judged 'least fit' and the other 'most fit.' During a three-month observation, 7 percent of the firefighters in the 'least fit' group suffered from back pain that was intense enough to make them miss work. That was ten times higher than the rate in the 'most fit' group.

"And the fit firefighters also recovered quicker and returned to work faster."

And So Is Regeneration

A team of researchers at the University of Copenhagen showed that exercise could reverse as well as prevent. They took 105 chronic back pain sufferers and broke them into three different groups for three months. The participants rated their pain, disability, and physical impairment before treatment, at the end of treatment, and three months after the treatment had stopped.

One group tried hot compresses and back massage in combination with gentle isometric exercises that emphasized the spinal area.

Another group participated in 30 sessions of intensive back-strengthening exercises that lasted 1½ hours each time.

The third group worked out for as long as the second group, but performed their exercises at only one-fifth the intensity.

The best results—at the end of treatment *and* three months later—were reported by group two—the ones who sweated through the intensive exercise.

Pump Away Your Pain

What kind of exercise routine does Dr. Brown recommend? "One that involves tightening of the abdominal muscles and arching the back to strengthen the back muscles," he says. "It's a very simple program that most people in normal health can get right into.

"Nautilus or similar weight-training machines are good if people are taught to use them properly. I suggest warming up first for 5 to 10 minutes on a stationary bike. Then do a circuit of several machines, making sure to emphasize exercises that help the stomach and back muscles. After you're done, do some stretching exercises. The workout should take about 45 minutes and should be repeated three times a week."

(But *first*, says Dr. Brown, make sure you get your back checked out. *Most* lower back pain is due to poor posture, smoking, and an overweight out-of-shape owner; but you should be certain that yours isn't something more serious, like arthritis or a disk gone bad. Once you get the all-clear signal from a medical professional, you can work that back, back into shape—safely.)

And that workout program is a much healthier prescription, says Dr. Brown, than what physicians recommended a generation ago.

"In the old days," he explains, "people were put into traction for long periods of time and given muscle relaxants, painkillers, and sleeping pills. Not infrequently, all that lying in bed actually *increased* the pain. And, of course, we know that you shouldn't take painkillers for long periods of time.

"The treatments very much contributed to the problem, and after a while, the doctor and the patient would get so frustrated that exploratory surgery would be performed."

And such surgery is often a bigger mistake than the pills and bed rest.

So if your doctor starts writing you a prescription for the same kind of pills that some people sell on the street (or suggests that you sleep on that bad back for a week), consider seeking a second opinion from an enlightened practitioner like Dr. Brown—one who feels that "the best way to treat people is to guide them into good health practices."

The Stress Factor

You work in a pressure cooker. The tension mounts as the day wears on, and you say you can literally feel the pain building up in the small of your back.

Sorry, but the American Academy of Orthopaedic Surgeons says that stress does not *cause* lower back pain. But they add that if you have a back problem to begin with, stress can definitely aggravate the situation.

An emotionally upset or stressed person is often very tense, explains the academy. If they already have back problems, that tension increases the likelihood of muscle spasms in their back. Those spasms lead to pain, which, of course, causes the muscles to tighten up even more. It's the old vicious circle.

No, stress alone can't cause an aching back. But it *is* right there in the wings, ready and willing to make the problem worse.

Another way that stress can cause problems, adds Dr. Brown, is when people respond to it badly. Nothing wipes away stress like a good workout, but some people seem to have missed that message.

"These people have fallen into a nonexercise response to stress," he observes. "Often they wind down after a hard day with a few drinks, and then go to bed. Then, on the weekend, they'll grab a tennis racquet. In their weakened condition, they're prime candidates for lower back trouble.

"If they had worked out instead of sacked out, they'd have a back less likely to be injured when they play hard on the weekend. And they'd probably play a much better game, as well."

Read about It, Hear about It, Watch It

The American Academy of Orthopaedic Surgeons (AAOS) offers a free brochure on the problem of lower back pain and treatment options. You can get one by sending a stamped, self-addressed envelope to: Low Back Pain, AAOS, P.O. Box 618, Park Ridge, IL 60068.

Art Ulene, the TV doctor (did you know that he's a gynecologist, by the way?), got together with a committee of the AAOS and produced a "Back Pain Relief" program that's available on videotape or as an audiocassette.

Both include an exercise program designed to prevent pain, strengthen your back, and increase flexibility. There are also guidelines on how to use your back properly, and relaxation techniques that relieve the effects of stress and reduce tension.

You can order either by calling (800) 621-1203. The audio tape will set you back $9.95; ask for item 0–394–56082–5. The video costs $29.95; it's item 0–932513–27–1. Both come with an instructional booklet.

Tips for Cool Summer Walking

When the dog days of August start closing in, heat and humidity may make your walking program look like pure tomfoolery. It's tempting then to think of calling it quits till the autumn breezes woo you out again.

It's no joke. Heat and humidity can dampen more than just your spirits. They do stress your body. But there's no need to stop and give up all the conditioning you've gained so far. Here are some suggestions for reducing the risks of summer heat or finding temporary alternate routes for walking to fitness.

No-Sweat Walking

Talk with your doctor. If you have a specific health problem that makes walking outdoors in high temperatures unhealthy for you, or you just find it too darn uncomfortable to be outside, then do what thousands of Americans are doing—head for the malls. And we don't mean for a shopping spree or an ice-cream soda.

Malls across the country are opening their doors to walkers before the stores open. You can walk to your heart's content (and ease) in a temperature- and humidity-controlled environment.

Be forewarned: Mallwalkers take their walking seriously. You'll find everyone from strollers to racewalkers perambulating on these indoor courses.

Be careful of wet, slippery surfaces on rainy days. Many malls have varying textured surfaces now, rather than endless linoleum. According to podiatrist Richard J. Robinson, D.P.M., of Santa Paula, California, the change in the terrain of the floor makes your feet and legs use different muscles and you tire less quickly.

Indoor tracks at the local Y are a good bet, too, although they tend to be less temperature controlled than the malls.

Water Walking

You can totally immerse yourself in this method of walking. Stay cool in the pool but get your exercise by walking in thigh- to chest-high water. The potential benefits are the same as walking on land but with less sweat and lower risk of injury. The water supports the body's weight, making this an ideal exercise for people with weight problems or arthritis. Unlike swimming, you can walk and talk with your pool partner while you exercise, which may banish the boredom factor of doing laps across the pool.

Your local Y may have a water-walking program. Or you can walk in an outdoor pool. Of course, you'll need to slather on the sunscreen if you're going to be water walking outside.

Experts suggest that if you walk in chest-high water, try swinging your arms in the water for a total body workout. Start walking very slowly for the first few minutes and then try to reach a speed that feels vigorous without being exhausting. And don't forget to include a cool-down period!

Staying Cool Outdoors

If walking outside is your passion, there are lots of things you can do to help yourself withstand the hot weather:

• Wear a breathable hat to keep the sun off your head and face. A terry-cloth hat that you can soak in water is ideal. It can cool your head and block the sun's rays. Visors are okay, but the top of your head may feel hot. Hats that don't breathe trap heat in.

• Wear light, loose clothing. Heat loss occurs through the evaporation of sweat from your skin. The more skin exposed to the air, the more heat is lost. Wear as little as possible, but again, protect your skin with sunscreen.

• Drink plenty of water. Unless you're water walking, it's better to put the water in your body rather than on it. Carry a plastic water bottle and drink periodically on your walk (sometimes thirst is a delayed reaction) or plan stops near water sources. Avoid sugary drinks. Sugar prevents the stomach from emptying and delays water to the tissues.

• Walk early in the morning or in the early evening. This avoids the steamiest temperatures and most skin-scorching rays.

• Don't go out when the weather is very hot and steamy. You risk heatstroke or heat exhaustion. If humidity is low and there's a good breeze, warm-weather workouts should be safe.

• Beware of sudden fluctuations in temperature. If you're traveling from a cooler climate to a warmer one for vacation, be careful. It takes the body about 10 to 14 days to adjust to heat and humidity. Take it extra slow.

Feet Facts

Sidewalks are heating up and the temperature inside your shoes is soaring. That can mean more sweat, more blisters, athlete's foot, and infections.

Be sure to change your socks often and consider using an antifungal foot powder. Switch to a lighter shoe with lots of ventilation. Leather shoes can be ventilated by your shoemaker by punching air holes around the arch to make air rush in as you step.

All about Moisturizers

People ask more questions about moisturizers than about any other skin-care product. So *Prevention* consulted the professionals—cosmetic chemists and dermatologists— to answer these frequently asked questions. Here's what they said.

How can I get the best results from a moisturizer for dry, sensitive skin?

"When buying a moisturizer, look for the words 'non-acnegenic' or 'noncomedogenic' on the label," says Wilma Bergfeld, M.D., a dermatologist at the Cleveland Clinic Foundation. "That means it won't clog your pores.

"Also, try nonallergenic or hypoallergenic products," she says. "Manufacturers of these products have taken out the ingredients that typically cause allergic reactions."

If you have sensitive skin, don't use products that contain preservatives, perfumes, or colors. These are the three most irritating categories of ingredients.

It's especially important for people with very dry skin to use a moisturizer both in the morning and after bathing. "The worst thing you can do for dry, sensitive skin is to hop out of a hot shower and then go straight outside," says Gary Grove, Ph.D., vice president of research and development at the KGL Skin Study Center in Broomall, Pennsylvania. Using a moisturizer right after bathing or showering seals in your skin's moisture. If you don't use one within half an hour, the water on your skin will evaporate, taking some of your skin's natural oil with it.

I see the terms "microsphere" and "microencapsulation" in a lot of moisturizer ads. I'm confused. What do they mean?

These terms are used differently by each company. Basically, both microsphere and microencapsulation mean that the moisturizer's active ingredients are contained in tiny bubbles or spheres.

This technology has been used in timed-release drug-delivery systems. Now cosmetic chemists have adapted microencapsulation to deliver timed-release emollients. "These microspheres are porous and can be loaded with the active ingredient," explains Sergio Nacht, Ph.D., senior vice president of research and development at Advanced Polymer Systems. "Not only do you get the ingredient over time, but as you rub your skin, ingredients are released on demand."

More recently, cosmetic chemists have also adapted this technology to help improve an ingredient's penetration to the deeper layers of your skin. The stratum corneum, your skin's outermost layer, normally functions as a protective barrier against germs. But this layer can also act as a barrier to moisturizers. "There's good reason to believe that by having the active ingredients penetrate deeper, you'll get a longer-lasting effect," adds Dr. Grove.

I've seen vitamin E acetate in moisturizers. What does it do?

Studies of vitamin E acetate are relatively new, and there's some controversy over its importance.

Basically, vitamin E is a very good natural moisturizer with antioxidant properties. This means it has the ability to neutralize free radicals, certain chemical compounds formed in the body that damage the skin cells. Vitamin E acetate protects your skin by trapping free radicals.

"Anti-aging skin preparations should routinely include both vitamin E acetate and a sunscreen," says cosmetic chemist Charles Fox, a consultant to the cosmetics industry. "If we can reduce the free radicals, we can delay the aging process a bit." Using vitamin E from capsules meant to be swallowed, however, is not recommended.

Can my moisturizer go bad if I buy it in large quantities?

There are three potential problems with buying moisturizers in one big jar. The first is rancidity. Some of the oils used in moisturizers are very rich in polyunsaturates, which go rancid quickly. As long as the container is closed, the product will stay fresh. But once it's open, you should use up the moisturizer within a month or two, or it will go bad. (You'll know because it will smell "off.") You can help preserve your product by keeping the container tightly closed between uses so oxygen can't get in.

The second problem is contamination. You should always wash your hands before putting your fingers in the bottle or jar. If you don't, you'll be introducing microbes into the product, and moisturizers offer a rich environment in which germs can multiply.

The last problem is separation. "Moisturizers remain effective indefinitely (even if they turn rancid) because they don't decompose," says Fox. Still, since most moisturizers are emulsions, which are mixtures of oil and water, the ingredients may separate. If that happens, all you have to do is shake it. The product may look funny, but the chemicals will stay intact.

Do moisturizers lose effectiveness if your skin gets used to them?

Not to the best of our knowledge. In fact, a good way to eliminate dryness is by frequent applications of a moisturizer. Once the problem is under control, you can apply a lighter moisturizer or use the same product less often.

No matter how much moisturizer I use, my skin still looks red and chapped. What else can I do?

You might want to see your dermatologist. According to Dr. Bergfeld, people often mistake the red, flaky skin of an early stage of seborrheic dermatitis for simple dry skin. This is especially true when this condition occurs on the face. "Plain dry skin is not red," explains Dr. Bergfeld. "Redness often indicates a condition such as seborrheic dermatitis—inflammatory dandruff of the skin."

A dermatologist will be able to diagnose and treat conditions that a moisturizer alone can't help.

What kind of tests do moisturizers have to pass before they're put on the market?
Current laws don't specify any standards for moisturizers. Still, the major companies do extensive testing through their own and independent laboratories to substantiate claims for a new product. Much of the impetus for such testing comes from the increasingly refined wants of both consumers and dermatologists. Doctors are seeing more and more people with good complexions who want to retard aging and seek recommendations on which brands to use to treat specific problems. The shift toward preventive maintenance has created a need for products that live up to their claims.

The Dermatology Foundation, a nonprofit organization, is in the process of developing a seal of approval based on meaningful criteria for certain dermatologic products. The standards are expected to go into effect within the next couple of years.

Special Supplement

Quick Fixes

It often seems that nothing takes just 1 minute. Probably even the "Minute Waltz" runs at least 65 seconds, if not longer. What, then, can you possibly do to improve your health in 1 minute? Well, as a result of checking scientific studies and consulting medical experts, *Prevention* found many remedies that you can apply in nothing flat to dozens of common ills.

Almost all these techniques take about a minute to do (although a few must be repeated several times before the problem is cured). Some may take only a minute to work; some, only a few seconds. Most, much longer. Many can be done at home, but there are also a few lesser-known tricks that only a doctor should perform.

Many remedies on this list have been scientifically tested—as close to sure things as possible. Others are simply shortcuts recommended by physicians. And some are just healing possibilities based on the educated guesses of researchers.

So allowing for a few seconds either way, here's a catalog of the world's fastest therapies.

Soothing the Skin

1. Moisturizing Skin • Add a glassful of ordinary milk to your bath water to soothe dry skin. Proteins in milk help soften and moisturize. (Bathing in water with a cupful of salt added works, too, though you have to rinse off the salt water afterward.) Apply lotion after bathing while the skin is still damp.

2. Beating Bug Bites • To relieve the itch of mosquito or other insect bites, apply a paste of baking soda and water. The alkaline moisture soothes irritation.

3. Easing Bee Stings • Minimize the pain of bee stings with a dash of papain, an enzyme in meat tenderizers like Adolph's or McCormick. (Accent has no papain.) First, gently flick out the stinger with a fingernail or file, then briefly apply ice or dunk in cold water. Apply a thin paste of tenderizer and water. Papain destroys the venom in the sting. (If you're allergic to bee stings, or if you start to have a reaction—hives or difficulty breathing—see a doctor immediately!)

4. Neutralizing Jellyfish "Close Encounters" • Jellyfish stings are aggravated by washing with fresh water. The best thing you can do is neutralize the toxins by soaking the area of the sting in one of three liquids: alcohol, vinegar, or a solution of papain-containing meat tenderizer and salt water. Then apply a paste of flour, talc, or baking soda dissolved in salt water. (If the pain doesn't go away in a few hours, or you have muscle pains, nausea, or signs of shock, call a doctor.)

5. Slipping Out Slivers • A little vegetable oil can help you remove painful splinters. Just pat some on and wait a moment for it to seep around and into the puncture. Then gently remove the splinter with tweezers. The "lube job" should help it slide right out.

6. Peeling Away Microsplinters • Splinters that are too small to get with tweezers can be removed with white glue or facial mask gel. Pour a thin layer of glue or gel over the skin and let it dry. Then peel the dried glue/mask off. The splinters go with it! This trick has worked for wood splinters, fiberglass fragments, and even cactus spines.

7. Taking the Burn out of Sunburn • Soothe away sunburn pain with a cool or tepid oatmeal bath. There are several commercial brands of oatmeal bath soaks in the drugstore. Don't use your breakfast oatmeal—the flakes are too large.

8. Treating a Broken Blister • The best way to treat an ordinary blister is to leave it alone. If it breaks on its own, wash the area with soap and water and cover with a bandage. Minor burn blisters should be flushed with cold water. The fresh juice of an aloe vera plant can help speed healing. (For burns that cover a large area, see a doctor.)

9. Drying Out Sweaty Hands • Troubled by chronically perspiring palms? There is help, but it's available only through your doctor. A prescription drug with aluminum chloride (one brand name is Drysol) can be dabbed onto your hands and left overnight. (You'll have to cover your hands with clear plastic wrap and gloves, too.) Once perspiration is under control, the treatment can be done one night a week to maintain its effect.

10. Easing the Itching • To control itching from bug bites or minor poison ivy, alter the surface temperature of the rash with cold water. Drape a cold washcloth over the area for a few moments. Relief can last 3 hours.

11. Washing Away Poison Ivy • To prevent a rash from developing after exposure to poison oak, ivy, or sumac, run lots of cold water over the area that was exposed. This works especially well within 3 minutes or so after contact. There's no need to use soap, but a rubbing-alcohol rinse before using water is ideal. (Wash clothes that touched the plants, too.)

12. Soothing Canker Sores • Tincture of myrrh (an herb) is an old-time remedy for canker sores. Just apply a little on the center of the sore to reduce pain and promote healing. You can find myrrh at some health food stores and older neighborhood druggists. It's an ingredient in many commercial compounds, too.

13. Soothing Canker Sores, Part 2 • Dissolve an antacid tablet in your mouth. It neutralizes digestive juices that aggravate the sores.

14. Pickling Athlete's Foot • Fight chronic athlete's foot with this 1-minute-to-prepare soak. Fill a basin with warm water and add half a cup of white vinegar. This lowers the pH balance of your skin, making life uncomfortable for fungi and bacteria.

15. "Frying" Itchy Shingles • The painful skin condition known as shingles may be relieved instantly with a therapeutic cream made from capsaicin, the active ingredient in hot peppers. The cream is called Zostrix, and is available without a prescription.

16. Sticking It to Warts • A new stick-on pad containing salicylic acid is an easy way to treat warts. Put a pad over the wart each night, and take it off the next morning. It destroys most warts in four to eight weeks. The brand name is Trans-Ver-Sal, and it's available only by prescription. (Warning: People with poor circulation should not use these pads.)

17. Putting Warts in the Deep-Freeze • Dermatologists and podiatrists use a liquid nitrogen spray to freeze plantar warts (those on the bottom of the feet). They spray the wart for a few moments, and it falls off by itself within a few weeks.

18. Using the Cold-Toe Treatment • Doctors can also use liquid nitrogen for ingrown toenails. (This common ailment, by the way, is caused by skin growing over the nail, not by a piece of nail growing into the surrounding skin.) The infected skin is frozen in seconds, dies, and eventually peels away. And the nail is usually spared.

Wipe Out Aches and Pains

19. Curing a Charley Horse • Calf cramps can be massaged away: Grasp your toes and gently pull them toward you.

Use your other hand to rub lengthwise along the calf, from the back of the knee to the ankle. Always rub with the muscle, never across it.

20. Icing Hurt Muscles • Ice is the best emergency treatment for sprains and pulled muscles. But most of us don't have ice packs, and makeshift packs fall apart as the ice melts. Simple solution: Use a bag of frozen peas or other small vegetable. Bang it on the counter to break the peas apart, and it will conform to the contours of the injured area. Wrap it in a towel and leave on for no more than 20 minutes at a time.

21. Halting a Spasm • Overworked runners sometimes get side stitches, painful cramps probably caused by spasms of the diaphragm. The best way to get rid of these spasms is to slow down your pace and take slow, rhythmic breaths.

22. Numbing a Toothache • If you saw the movie *Marathon Man* and wondered if clove oil really works to relieve tooth pain, wonder no longer. It does. In fact, it's so powerful it can even damage nerves. So don't use the raw oil. Instead, find a commercial product with clove oil and use according to directions. Then see your dentist as soon as possible.

23. Beating Banged-Finger Syndrome • Ouch! Reduce the trauma by quickly immersing your finger in cold water. The pain is reduced almost immediately. It also helps keep swelling down, for less discomfort later.

24. Treating a Hangnail • Hangnails are not really slivers of hanging nail, but dried out and split skin along the nail's edge. And they can smart a lot. But rubbing a little petroleum jelly over and around them before you go to bed will ease the pain. How? The jelly will trap moisture and soften the dry skin underneath.

25. Rubbing Away Sinus Pain • Massaging the areas just under your eyebrows (and above the eyes) can help reduce or relieve some attacks of sinus pain. Make firm, slow circles with your thumbs or fingertips.

Ear, Nose, and Throat Soothers

26. Unclogging Your Ears • If you have allergies, you may sometimes get eustachian-tube blockage, which can cause the pain known as "allergic ear." But if your doctor approves, you can be ready with a fast remedy. The best way to relieve this pain is through the nose, with a strong decongestant spray, such as Neo-Synephrine. Tilt your head back and spray in enough decongestant through both nostrils so you can actually taste some of it in the back of your throat. This passes the drug directly over the opening to the eustachian tubes. (Caution: Nasal-decongestant sprays should not be used regularly or for chronic conditions without a doctor's supervision.)

27. Easing the Hurt of "High-Altitude Ear" • When yawning or chewing gum won't get rid of ear pain during airplane descent, try a modified Valsalva maneuver. Close your mouth, pinch your nose shut, and gently blow into your nose. This forces air into the middle ear to equalize pressure. You may hear a dull "pop." If you fly with a cold, try an oral decongestant. Warning: Heart patients should not try the Valsalva maneuver.

28. "Cupping" Unequal Ear Pressure • For severe ear pain that won't respond to the Valsalva maneuver, you may want to try this trick: Soak two washcloths in very hot water. Wring them out so they're saturated, but not dripping, and place each in a cup. Hold the cups over your ears. The steam heat seems to relax the eardrum.

29. Banishing Buzzing Bugs • If an insect flies into your ear, shine a light in the ear. Chances are, the critter will crawl back out toward the light. If it doesn't come out, it may be stuck in wax. If you're sure it's a bug, you can try to flush it out with water using a rubber ear bulb. If you're not sure it's a bug, don't flush the ear. Some substances absorb water, causing more problems. (For example, children sometimes stick pieces of food in their ears.) And don't go after the bug with a cotton swab. If these steps fail, call the doctor.

30. Unstuffing Your Nose • Adults occasionally suffer from a stuffy nose unrelated to allergies or colds. Doctors call it vasomotor rhinitis. It's caused by dilation of tiny blood vessels inside the nasal tissue. For instant, temporary relief, try an over-the-counter spray decongestant. If the problem doesn't clear up, it's probably not vasomotor rhinitis. Consult an allergist.

31. Curing a "Desert Nose" • A few squirts of saline solution up each nostril can rehydrate the mucous membranes of a dried-out nose. There are several commercial preparations available in drugstores. These products come in handy squirt bottles. Or make your own by mixing 1 teaspoon of salt with 2½ cups of warm water. Pour a small amount into your palm and inhale it into your nose.

32. Stanching a Nosebleed • If your nose is bleeding, sit down, lean forward, and hold both nostrils tightly shut for 15 minutes—no less! (Obviously, you'll breathe through your mouth.)

33. Dampening Down a Dry, Hacking Cough • Look for a cough-suppressant syrup or drops containing dextromethorphan. It's available in over 50 different products. (But don't take this drug if you've got asthma or chronic bronchitis. See a doctor if your cough persists for a few days.)

34. Quieting a Throat Tickle • Try this bitter but often effective cough remedy: Suck on a whole clove (the kind you stick in baked ham).

35. Soothing a Sore Throat • Perhaps the best thing to do for an ordinary sore throat is to gargle with warm salt water. The high salt concentration eases discomfort and may have a slight antibacterial action.

Vision Aids

36. Cooling Down Itchy Eyes • Close your eyes and cover them with cool cucumber slices for a few moments. A cool, wet washcloth can have the same effect.

37. "Watering" Dry Eyes • There are a number of good artificial-tear products on the market for occasional dry eyes. Here's a low-tech alternative: Soak a washcloth in warm to mildly hot water. Wring it out and put it over your eyes for a few minutes. The moist heat can unclog sluggish glands in the eyelids, inducing the eye to lubricate itself naturally.

38. Getting Around the Arid-Eye Syndrome • For people with Sjögren syndrome, dry eyes are a fact of life. But doctors can prescribe a lubricating pellet called Lacrisert. Inserted under the lower lid, it dissolves, lubricating the eye. One pellet usually lasts a full day.

39. Getting the Specks Out • If you get a speck in your eye, you may be able to wash it out with your own tears. Simply pull your upper lid downward, slightly over the lower lid. This will cause tears to flow. If that doesn't work, try flushing the eye with water. If irritation persists, see a doctor. These measures, of course, are effective only for tiny, movable specks. If the object is embedded in the eye, skip the self-care and get medical help right away.

40. Overcoming Eyestrain • If you do a lot of close work (reading, gazing at a computer screen, and the like), you may occasionally strain your eyes. To counteract this problem, take at least 1 full minute every hour or two and focus your gaze on a distant object.

41. Saving Sight with Light • Lasers can perform miracles in a few seconds. One of the most dramatic examples: Patients who've had cataract surgery can lose vision when the capsule around the lens clouds over (as happens in half of all cases). But a momentary zap of laser creates a shock wave that makes a tiny hole in the capsule. The patient is literally blind one minute and can see the next!

42. Taking Aim against Glaucoma • Glaucoma is a condition in which a pressure buildup inside the eye causes slow but serious damage. Unchecked, it can rob you of your sight. To control the condition, ophthalmologists perform an iridotomy—they make a tiny hole in the iris to drain excess fluid. This procedure used to be done in an operating room. Now it can be done in moments with a laser on an outpatient basis.

Internal Healing

43. Tilting against Heartburn • Heartburn is caused by leakage of digestive juices from the stomach into the esophagus. Lying down can aggravate the condition. But there's a solution for those who suffer heartburn at bedtime: Raise the head of the bed eight inches or so with blocks under the headboard. Caution: Recurrent heartburn should be checked by a physician.

44. Calming Indigestion • A cup of herbal tea made from peppermint, chamomile, or catnip can help quiet indigestion, says *Prevention* adviser Varro E. Tyler, Ph.D., in his book *The New Honest Herbal*. Note: In rare cases, some people experience a serious allergic reaction to certain herbal teas. For example, chamomile may cause problems for people allergic to ragweed.

45. Deterring Nausea • Powdered ginger may be more effective than Dramamine in preventing nausea and motion sickness. A study reported in *Lancet* tested the antinausea effect of three different treatments: two capsules of powdered ginger (940 milligrams total), a standard dose of Dramamine (100 milligrams), and two capsules of an inactive herb. The six test subjects who took ginger were able to stay in a revolving chair an average of 50 percent longer than the six on the drug. (The inactive-herb group fared much worse: Three of the six threw up.) Ginger is safe:

You can take two 450-milligram capsules (available in many health food stores) about 10 minutes before your flight or cruise, and two more again if you feel queasy.

46. Easing Occasional Constipation • Drink plain, hot water when you get up in the morning. The hot water seems to stimulate the natural movement of the intestinal tract. Since the intestines are usually active in the morning anyway, this remedy often works immediately. The water should be about as hot as your morning coffee or tea. Constipation that lasts more than five days, however, should be reported to your doctor.

More Relief

47. Blessing You and Your Back • Sneezing can be bad business for back pain sufferers and people with osteoporosis. The explosive force of a sneeze can actually cause injury to the structures of the spine. If you feel a sneeze coming, brace yourself by placing one hand on the front of your thigh or a table near you. If you're standing, you should also bend your knees.

48. Cooling a Singed Tongue • One of life's biggest little annoyances is a burned tongue. You may be able to ease the pain somewhat by sprinkling sugar on your tongue.

49. Sipping Some Asthma Relief • Drinking 18 ounces of strong coffee may relieve an asthma attack if you're caught without your asthma medication. Caffeine is chemically related to theophylline, a common asthma medication. Caffeine is not a good permanent substitute, though—it's only about 40 percent as potent.

50. Shrinking Hemorrhoids • Two warm baths per day can help soothe and shrink hemorrhoids. Apply hemorrhoid cream after the bath for maximum healing effect.

51. Warming Up Cold Hands • Swing your arms around in circles like a baseball pitcher doing warm-ups. This forces blood into your hands rapidly. The technique works for ordinary cold hands and for a disorder of the peripheral circulatory system called Raynaud's syndrome.

52. Slowing a Racing Heart • Tachycardia, or rapid heartbeat, can have many causes—not all of them unwanted. But paroxysmal atrial tachycardia is a disturbance of the natural rhythm of the heart. It can be controlled with drugs. A natural reaction called the diving reflex, though, may bring an attack under control in a few seconds. Simply fill a sink with cool water (about 65°F seems to work best). Breathe deeply a few times, then immerse your face in the water for 30 seconds (count "one thousand one, one thousand two," and so on). When you come up, the tachycardia should be under control. Warning: You should check with your doctor before trying this technique.

53. Tickling Away Hiccups • There must be hundreds of cures for hiccups, but only two have achieved mention in the *New England Journal of Medicine*. The first is to rub the roof of the mouth (at the point where hard and soft palate meet) with a cotton swab. This may overstimulate the nerve that triggers hiccups, causing it to shut down.

54. Sweetening the Hiccup Problem • The second *New England Journal of Medicine* hiccup cure is this: Swallow a spoonful of white sugar. Allow the granules to trickle down the back of your throat. Nerve endings there are overstimulated by the granules, interrupting the spasms.

55. Breathing Easier (Temporarily) • People with emphysema or asthma may be able to relieve breathlessness in the following position: Sit down and lean forward, with your elbows or hands on your knees. This compresses the abdomen and stretches the diaphragm upward, which can make breathing more effective.

56. Sugaring a Little Wound • You have a nasty cut, and you're out of first-aid cream. Simple solution: Pack the wound with sugar or honey. Microorganisms can't survive in concentrated solutions of sugar. This healing technique has been used for centuries.

57. Giving Bad Breath the Brush-Off • Brushing your tongue as well as your teeth can bring some cases of bad breath under control. One researcher found that this method reduced malodorous gases in exhaled breath by 85 percent. Of course, it doesn't work for bad breath caused by severe tooth decay.

58. Counting Out Panic Attacks • People with phobias are taught to cope with panic attacks in a number of ways. A common trick is distraction—taking your mind off the object of fear. One good method of distraction, according to president of the Phobia Society of America Jerilyn Ross, is to count backward from 100 by threes. If you get too good at it, try going backward from 150 by sevens.

59. Blowing Off Anxiety • The next time you feel tense, try the six-three-six method of instant relaxation: Inhale slowly through your nose for a count of six. Gently hold your breath for a count of three. Then exhale for a count of six. Repeat several times. Rhythmic breathing can sometimes short-circuit the fight-or-flight response during stressful situations.

Index

Boldface references indicate tables.

Rodale Press, Inc., publishes PREVENTION, America's leading health magazine. For information on how to order your subscription, write to PREVENTION, Emmaus, PA 18098.